EDINBURGH LONDON MADRID MELBOURNE NEW YORK AND TOKYO 1997

CHURCHILL LIVINGSTONE
Medical Division of Pearson Professional Limited

Distributed in the United States of America by
Churchill Livingstone Inc., 650 Avenue of the
Americas, New York, N.Y. 10011, and by
associated companies, branches and
representatives throughout the world.

First published as Colour Aids Orthopaedics 1986
First Colour Guide edition 1992
Second Colour Guide edition 1997

ISBN 0443 05806 7

British Library Cataloguing in Publication Data
A catalogue record for this book is available from
the British Library.

Library of Congress Cataloging in Publication Data
A catalog record for this book is available from
the Library of Congress.

Medical knowledge is constantly
changing. As new information
becomes available, changes in
treatment, procedures, equipment
and the use of drugs become
necessary. The author and the
publishers have, as far as it is
possible, taken care to ensure
that the information given in this
text is accurate and up to date.
However, readers are strongly
advised to confirm that the
information, especially with
regard to drug usage, complies
with current legislation and
standards of practice.

The
publisher's
policy is to use
**paper manufactured
from sustainable forests**

Produced by Longman Asia Limited,
Hong Kong SWTC/01

For Churchill Livingstone

Publisher: Michael Parkinson
Project Editor: James Dale
Project controller: Nancy Arnott
Design direction: Erik Bigland

Acknowledgements

I wish to thank colleagues who have generously provided illustrations: Mr J. Chalmers (Figs 80, 81, 89); Mr A. Gibson (Figs 114, 115); Professor P. J. Gregg (Figs 45, 167, 192); Professor S. P. F. Hughes (Figs 2, 48, 49, 51, 54, 76, 77, 100, 174, 179); Mr M. R. H. Khan (Figs 37, 38, 39); Mr D. W. Lamb (Fig. 132); Mr M. J. McMaster (Figs 23, 102); Mr M. F. Macnicol (Figs 29, 73, 159); Mr J. E. Phillips (Fig. 7); Mr J. E. Robb (Figs 32, 82); Mr J. H. Scott (Figs 110, 111); Mr R. K. Strachan (Fig. 173).

I am also grateful to Professor Hughes for allowing me to use slides from the collection in the Department of Orthopaedic Surgery, University of Edinburgh (Figs 1, 16, 33, 34, 57, 58, 59, 94, 97, 178, 196).

I thank Michael Devlin and Sonia Miller for their help in the preparation of photographic material and Alison McGowan for her assistance with the manuscript.

G.H.
Edinburgh

Contents

Acute osteomyelitis

Infection of bone caused by pyogenic bacteria (most commonly staphylococci or streptococci).

Pathology

Bacteria may enter the bone directly, e.g. from an open fracture, or via the blood stream from a septic focus elsewhere in the body. In the latter (haematogenous) type of osteomyelitis the infection usually occurs in the metaphysis of a long bone. Untreated infection causes thrombosis of blood vessels and death of bone. An abscess may form under the periosteum.

Clinical features

Haematogenous osteomyelitis usually affects children. There is a fairly rapid onset with malaise, pyrexia and pain over the affected part. Examination reveals local warmth and tenderness. Erythema (Fig. 1) may be present but is absent in the early stages.

Investigations

ESR is raised. The infecting organism may be identified by culturing blood withdrawn before antibiotics are started.

Radiographs are initially negative but later a subperiosteal reaction may be seen (Fig. 2). An isotope bone scan is positive at an early stage (Fig. 3).

Treatment

Early stage. Rest, fluid replacement and broad spectrum antibiotics in high dosage pending identification of the organism.

Later stage. Surgical drainage is necessary if there is no response to appropriate antibiotics, or if an abscess has formed.

Complications

Septicaemia, chronic osteomyelitis (p. 3), septic arthritis (p. 3), and damage to growth plate causing deformity in growing bone.

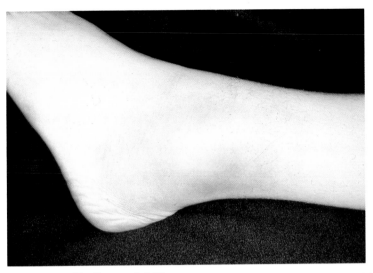

Fig. 1 Osteomyelitis of lower end of tibia.

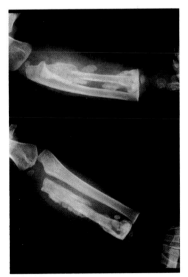

Fig. 2 Untreated acute osteomyelitis of the radius showing vigorous periosteal reaction.

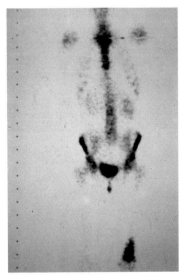

Fig. 3 Bone scan showing increased uptake at lower end of left femur.

Chronic osteomyelitis

Chronic infection of bone. It usually follows an episode of acute osteomyelitis that has not been treated adequately.

Pathology

The bone is thickened and filled with granulation tissue. Fragments of dead bone (sequestra) are often present. Pus may discharge through sinuses leading from the bone to the skin surface (Fig. 4).

Clinical features

Pain, intermittent discharge of pus and, rarely, malignant change in a sinus. A sequestrum may be visible on a radiograph (Fig. 5).

Treatment

Very difficult. Appropriate antibiotics will control flare-ups of infection. A sinus may heal after removal of a sequestrum, but for permanent cure all dead and infected material must be removed.

Septic arthritis

Bacterial infection of a joint, usually by the pyogenic organisms that cause acute osteomyelitis. When the metaphysis of a long bone is intracapsular (e.g. the proximal metaphyses of the femur and humerus), bacteria from a focus of osteomyelitis may infect the joint. Septic arthritis may also be due to haematogenous spread of bacteria or direct entry through a wound.

Clinical features

Pyrexia and malaise. The affected joint is swollen, tender and warm. Radiographs are normal at first. Later there is periarticular osteoporosis followed by joint destruction (Fig. 6).

Treatment

Rest, splintage and antibiotics. Surgical drainage rather than aspiration of the joint is usually necessary and should be done early since articular cartilage does not regenerate after it has been damaged.

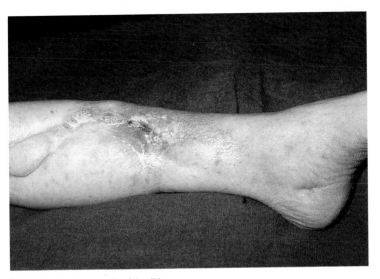

Fig. 4 Chronic osteomyelitis of the tibia.

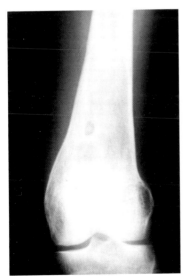

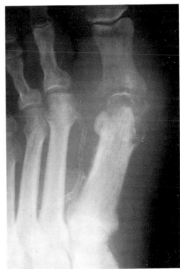

Fig. 5 A small sequestrum in the lower part of the femur.

Fig. 6 Destruction of the metatarsophalangeal joint due to septic arthritis in a diabetic patient.

Tuberculosis

Bones and joints can be infected by one of the various types of tubercle bacilli. Infection can occur at any age. The tubercle bacilli enter bone via the blood stream or by direct spread from another focus.

Clinical features

The patient is usually unwell with the general signs of tuberculosis, e.g. weight loss, pyrexia, night sweats.

Specific features depend on the site of infection. Large joints and the spine are most often affected but small bones in the hand can be involved (dactylitis).

Large joints. There is pain, swelling and limitation of movement. The muscles around the joint are often wasted.

Spine. Destruction of the intervertebral disc and adjacent vertebrae may cause a kyphosis (Fig. 7). Paraplegia may be a feature. Tuberculous pus may track down from the spine to form an abscess in the groin (a psoas abscess).

Investigations

Mantoux test is positive. ESR is raised during active infection.

Radiographs may show a paravertebral abscess in spinal infection (Fig. 8) or destruction of an affected joint (Fig. 9). A biopsy of the affected area will show the histological features of tuberculosis and allow culture of infected material.

Treatment

Rest and splintage of the affected joint, antituberculous chemotherapy and arthrodesis of painful unstable joints.

Surgical drainage and stabilization of spinal lesions may be indicated, particularly if there are neurological signs or a progressive kyphosis.

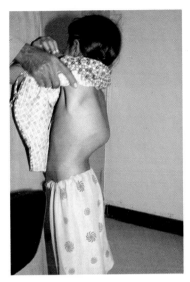

Fig. 7 Tuberculous kyphosis.

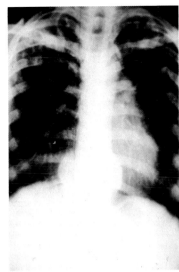

Fig. 8 Paravertebral abscess seen behind heart shadow.

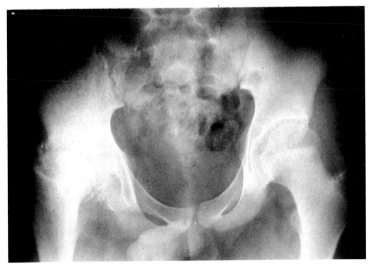

Fig. 9 Tuberculous destruction of the right hip.

Osteoarthritis

A common condition due to 'wear and tear' of joints. It may be primary (idiopathic) or secondary to any condition that causes damage or irregularity of the joint surface, such as injury, avascular necrosis (p. 45), osteochondritis dissecans (p. 125), Perthes' disease (p. 111) or septic arthritis (p. 3).

Synonyms

Osteoarthrosis; degenerative arthritis; OA.

Clinical features

More common with advancing age. Affected joints are painful and stiff and may become deformed.
   Primary OA may affect several joints but secondary OA tends to occur in one major weight bearing joint such as the hip or knee.

Investigations

The radiological features are loss of joint space, sclerosis of subchondral bone, osteophytes and cysts (Fig. 10).

Treatment

Analgesics. Physiotherapy often eases symptoms. Walking aids may be helpful. Obese patients should lose weight.
   Surgical treatment may be indicated if these general measures are not effective. The main types of operation are:

Arthrodesis. Surgical fusion of a joint (Fig. 11). Used mainly in small joints as arthrodesis of the hip or knee may be disabling despite good pain relief.

Osteotomy. Realignment of a joint by cutting through adjacent bone (Fig. 12). Effective in correcting deformity but pain relief is unpredictable.

Excision arthroplasty. Surgical removal of a joint (Fig. 13). Not used as a primary procedure in large joints.

Replacement arthroplasty. See page 9. ➡

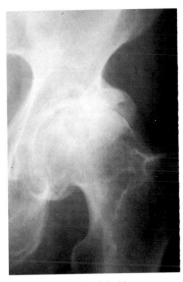

Fig. 10 Osteoarthritis of the hip.

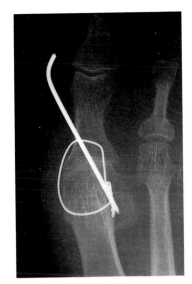

Fig. 11 Arthrodesis of the first metatarsophalangeal joint.

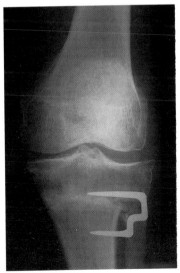

Fig. 12 Upper tibial osteotomy for OA of knee.

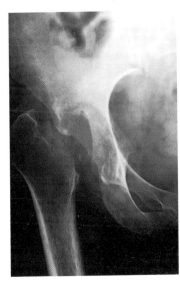

Fig. 13 Excision arthroplasty of hip.

Total joint replacement. The affected joint is excised and an artificial joint is inserted. Replacements have been designed for many joints but are most successful in the hip and, to a lesser extent, the knee.

An ideal artificial joint must be stable and anatomically similar to the structure it replaces. It must be made of materials that are biologically inert, have low friction characteristics and are not prone to wear. Typically the joint is made of a metal, such as stainless steel, and high molecular weight polyethylene (Fig. 14) since these materials have generally satisfactory properties. The components are stabilized in position with methylmethacrylate cement (Fig. 15). Many other materials such as titanium, chrome–cobalt alloys and ceramics are in use or under evaluation, as are joints that do not require stabilization by cement.

Complications

A successful joint replacement relieves pain and often improves movement but complications are not uncommon and tend to increase with time after the operation.

Infection (Fig. 16) causes painful loosening. Exchange arthroplasty is technically difficult and not always successful. Removal of the joint may be necessary, resulting in an excision arthroplasty (Fig. 13).

Mechanical failure of the components can occur (Fig. 17).

In addition a prosthetic joint may *dislocate* or *heterotopic ossification* may occur around it, resulting in loss of movement.

See also osteoarthritis of spine (p. 75), hand (p. 103), hip (p. 115), knee (p. 127) and foot (p. 145).

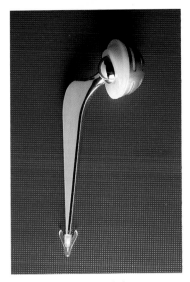

Fig. 14 Femoral and acetabular components of a total hip replacement.

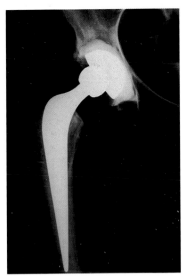

Fig. 15 Radiograph of a total hip replacement.

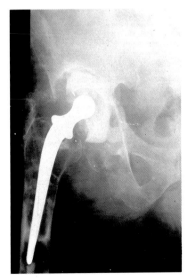

Fig. 16 An infected, loose, hip replacement.

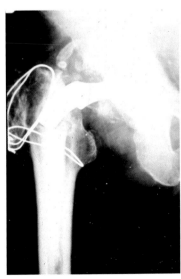

Fig. 17 Mechanical failure of the stem of the femoral component.

Rheumatoid arthritis

A common polyarthritis characterized by proliferation of the synovial lining of joints.

Cause

Unknown. An immunological basis seems likely.

Pathology

A chronic proliferative synovitis that causes stretching of joint capsules and ligaments, rupture of tendons and eventual destruction of articular cartilage.

Clinical features

Women are more often affected than men. Usual age of onset is 20–60 years, although juvenile forms do occur. Morning stiffness, pain and swelling are prominent features. Small joints of the hands and feet are usually affected first in a symmetrical fashion but occasionally one large joint, such as the knee, is involved initially.

On examination the affected joints are warm and erythema may be a feature. Synovial thickening is palpable in joints or around tendons (Fig. 18). Rheumatoid nodules are classically found on the extensor aspect of the forearm near the elbow (Fig. 19) but are not always present.

The natural history of the disease is very variable, ranging from a transient attack with recovery to the rapid development of severe, crippling deformities.

Investigations

ESR is raised in active phase. RA latex test is positive in some patients.

The first radiographic change is periarticular osteoporosis. Erosions are characteristic—small 'bites' from bones adjacent to joints, best seen in the metacarpophalangeal or metatarsophalangeal joints (Fig. 20). Loss of joint space, bone destruction and deformity are later features. ➡

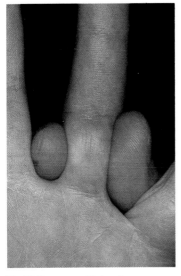

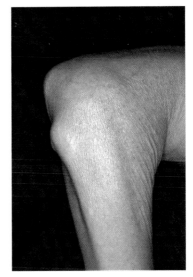

Fig. 18 Flexor synovitis in a finger.

Fig. 19 A rheumatoid nodule.

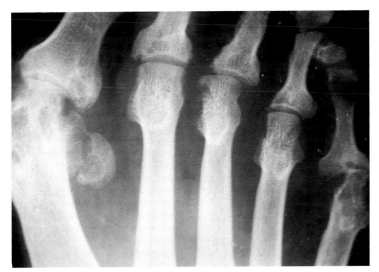

Fig. 20 Periarticular erosions in the foot.

Course	The initial episode may settle, leaving little functional disability, but further attacks may occur. In most patients the disease is chronic with exacerbations but may eventually 'burn out'. Progressive destruction of joints in the hands (Fig. 21), feet (Fig. 22) or major weight bearing joints produces severe disability.
Treatment	Relief of pain by anti-inflammatory drugs and rest in splints, provision of appliances to help with activities of daily living, and social support, including help with appropriate employment.

Surgical treatment

Surgical treatment is indicated mainly in patients with severe disability and deformity. A combined assessment by rheumatologist, orthopaedic surgeon, occupational therapist and physiotherapist is essential before surgery is advised. Surgery is planned to provide maximal functional benefit to the patient. Several operations may be necessary and their timing and sequence require careful planning.

The general types of surgical procedure are:

Soft tissue repairs. For example repair of ruptured tendons.

Synovectomy. Removal of involved synovium. Now rarely done on joints although diseased synovium may be removed from around tendons.

Arthrodesis (p. 7). Particularly for small joints in hand, wrist and ankle.

Arthroplasty (p. 9). Excision arthroplasty is used in the forefoot and replacement arthroplasty in the hip and knee.

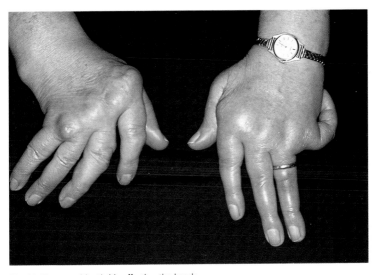

Fig. 21 Rheumatoid arthritis affecting the hands.

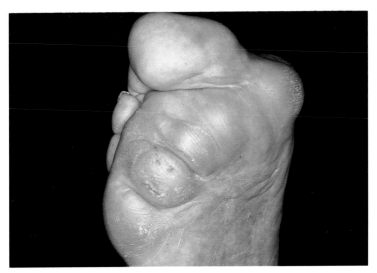

Fig. 22 Severe rheumatoid changes in the forefoot.

Ankylosing spondylitis

A chronic inflammatory disorder, typically affecting the spine and sacroiliac joints, which leads to ossification of ligaments. Fairly common (about 1 in 200 men but less often affects women).

Clinical features

Onset is between 18 and 30 years.

Early. Low back pain which typically wakens the patient in the morning. Stiffness of peripheral joints occurs in about 10%. Common clinical findings are limitation of spinal movement and chest expansion.

Late. Without treatment there is a tendency for the spine and affected joints to become stiffer. Progressive kyphosis can occur, making it difficult for the patient to see ahead (Fig. 23).

Investigations

ESR is raised in early active phase. HLA B27 antigen is present in 95% of patients. (This is *not a* diagnostic test since many unaffected people have the same antigen.)

Radiographs of the spine classically show calcification of the intervertebral ligaments, eventually producing the 'bamboo spine' (Fig. 24), but such changes should not be seen if treatment is early and vigorous. The sacroiliac joints are usually narrow and sclerotic (Fig. 25).

Treatment

Early. Active exercise programme to prevent stiffness, and anti-inflammatory analgesic drugs.

Late. Total hip replacement for stiff hips. Rarely, spinal osteotomy is indicated for severe deformity.

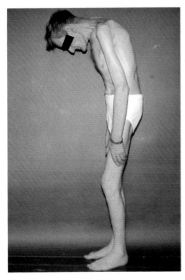

Fig. 23 Typical spinal deformity in severe ankylosing spondylitis.

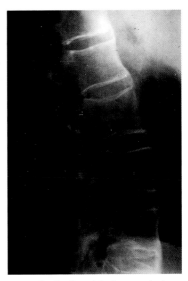

Fig. 24 Ossification of the intervertebral ligaments.

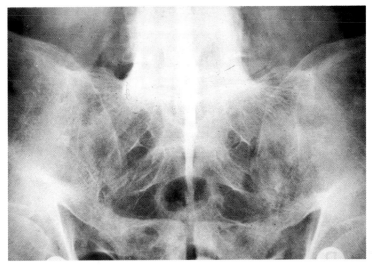

Fig. 25 Obliteration of the sacroiliac joints. Note ossification of the interspinous ligament.

Gout

A metabolic disorder characterized by hyperuricaemia and deposition of urate crystals around joints. It may be secondary to polycythaemia or myeloproliferative disorders, or precipitated by trauma (including surgery), dietary factors or certain drugs, notably diuretics.

More common in men. Usually one joint (typically the metatarsophalangeal joint of the big toe) is affected, with acute onset of severe pain, redness and swelling (Fig. 26). If untreated there will be recurrent attacks and eventually a chronic arthritis with deposition of urate tophi and damage to the joint (Fig. 27).

Serum urate is raised in acute attack. Characteristic crystals seen on microscopy of joint aspirate.

An acute attack is treated with anti-inflammatory drugs and further attacks are prevented by long-term treatment with uricosuric agents. Surgery to remove gouty tophi is rarely needed.

Chondrocalcinosis

Accumulation of crystals of calcium pyrophosphate within joints.

Pyrophosphate arthropathy; pseudogout.

Like gout, it occurs most often around 60 years, but the incidence is the same in men and women. One joint is affected, usually the knee. In the acute attack there is swelling, redness, pain, stiffness and an effusion within the joint.

Fluid aspirated from the joint is turbid and laden with leucocytes. Weakly birefringent crystals are seen under polarized light. Radiographs show calcification of intra-articular fibrocartilage (Fig. 28).

Anti-inflammatory analgesics.

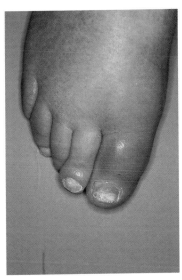

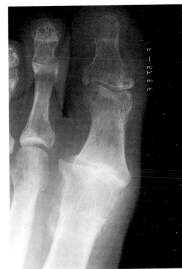

Fig. 26 Acute gout in the big toe.

Fig. 27 Gouty arthropathy in big toe.

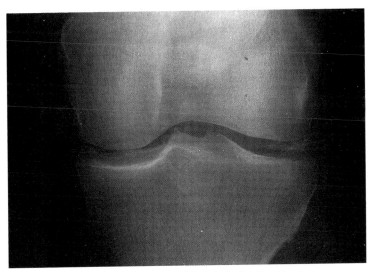

Fig. 28 Calcification of the lateral meniscus of the knee in chondrocalcinosis.

Haemophilic arthropathy

Haemophilia is a disorder of the blood-clotting mechanism due to deficiency of Factor VIII. It is transmitted as an X-linked recessive trait and therefore it nearly always affects males.

Clinical features

Recurrent haemarthroses (Fig. 29) cause painful swelling of joints and eventually produce a chronic arthropathy. The knees are most often involved but elbows, shoulders, wrists, ankles and hips may be affected. The joint involvement is usually asymmetrical. Radiographs are initially normal but later show a loss of joint space and a characteristic squaring of the articular region (Fig. 30).

Treatment

Immobilization, replacement of Factor VIII, analgesia, prevention of contractures by splinting. Joint replacement is sometimes necessary.

Psoriatic arthropathy

Occurs in 10% of people with psoriasis.

Clinical features

Skin disorder may not be marked. Many patients who develop arthritis have only thickening or pitting of the nails (Fig. 31). Arthritis can affect any joint, but typically attacks the small joints of the hands. Onset is sometimes acute, with erythema and swelling. Later features are similar to rheumatoid arthritis with sometimes severe destructive arthropathy affecting the hands and feet.

Treatment

Analgesic and anti-inflammatory drugs. Surgical arthrodesis of small joints may be indicated if pain and instability warrant it.

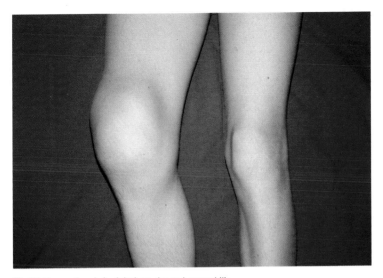

Fig. 29 Haemarthrosis in right knee due to haemophilia.

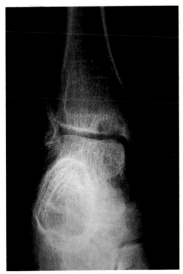

Fig. 30 Radiological changes in left ankle due to haemophilia.

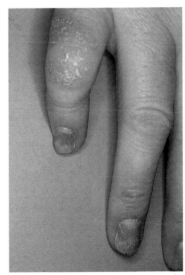

Fig. 31 Nail and skin changes in psoriatic arthropathy.

Cerebral palsy

Non-progressive brain damage affecting upper motor neurone function, often resulting in poor control of voluntary muscles.

Causes

Cerebral maldevelopment, fetal anoxia, birth trauma, infections and head injuries.

Incidence

Around 2 per 1000 children of school age.

Classification

By limbs affected: e.g. hemiplegia, diplegia (Fig. 32), quadriplegia.

By pattern of muscle dysfunction: Spastic (increased tone), athetoid (uncontrolled writhing movements), ataxic (poor coordination), rigid or mixed.

Clinical features

Varies with type of cerebral palsy. Locomotor disability is only one aspect; there may be mental deficiency, although this is not invariable. Associated disorders of speech, vision and hearing are also common.

Management

A team approach is important. The paediatrician, psychologist, physiotherapist, teacher and many other specialists will be involved in helping the child and family.

Orthopaedic aspects

Spasm of muscles causes limbs to be held in abnormal positions and fixed deformities may develop. Typical deformities are flexion of the elbow and wrist, adduction of hips, flexion of knees and plantar flexion (equinus) of foot (Fig. 33). Imbalance between spastic hip adductors and weak flexors may cause subluxation or even dislocation of the hip (Fig. 34).

Deformities can be minimized by muscle training, splintage and bracing. In carefully selected patients, operations such as tendon lengthening, tendon transfer, arthrodesis and muscle denervation may be useful.

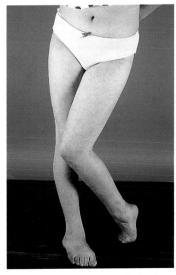

Fig. 32 Spastic diplegia in cerebral palsy.

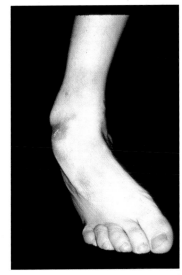

Fig. 33 Equinus and inversion deformity of foot.

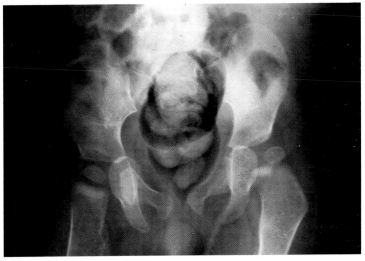

Fig. 34 Subluxation of left hip in a child with cerebral palsy.

Poliomyelitis

An infectious disease, usually affecting children, caused by one of the polioviruses which have an affinity for the cell bodies of motor neurones in the anterior horn of the spinal cord and brain stem. Can occur as an epidemic in an unvaccinated population.

Clinical features

The disease is mild in most cases, causing no more than a flu-like illness with gastrointestinal upset.

If the anterior horn cells are damaged, the muscles innervated by them will be paralysed. Paralysis may be partial or complete, temporary or permanent, depending on the extent and severity of neurological involvement.

The disease can be divided into five stages:
1. Incubation—14 days
2. Onset—2 days
3. Severe paralysis—around 2 months
4. Recovery of paralysis—up to 2 years
5. Residual paralysis—permanent.

Orthopaedic aspects

Total paralysis will render a limb flail. An appropriate orthosis for the leg will allow weight bearing.

Partial paralysis causes an imbalance in strength between groups of muscles acting on joints and this can lead to deformity, particularly in the growing child (Figs 35, 36).

Mobile deformities can be minimized by splinting, or tendon transfers to rebalance the muscles acting across a joint. Fixed deformities may require correction by osteotomy or arthrodesis of joints.

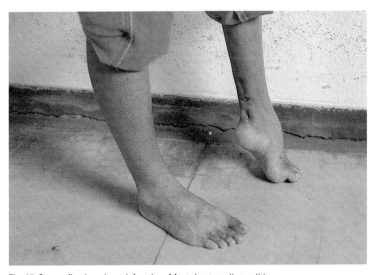

Fig. 35 Severe fixed equinus deformity of foot due to poliomyelitis.

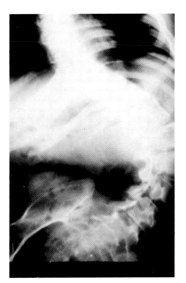

Fig. 36 A gross scoliosis due to imbalance of muscles acting on the spine.

Muscular dystrophies

Disorders in which there are primary pathological changes within muscles, usually giving rise to progressive weakness.

Types

Three examples will be given to illustrate some orthopaedic aspects of these conditions.

Pseudohypertrophic (Duchenne) muscular dystrophy. Transmitted as a sex-linked recessive characteristic and therefore affects boys. Onset aged 3–5 with weakness and a tendency to fall. The child 'climbs up his legs' to straighten up (Fig. 37) because of weakness in the hip extensors. Heel cords may become tight, causing equinus deformity of foot. Eventually the child is confined to a wheelchair and death from respiratory complications usually occurs towards the end of the second decade.

Congenital myopathies. Various types are recognized; typical features are 'floppiness' in babies and weakness in young children. Orthopaedic features include dislocation of the hip (p. 107), flat feet (p. 135) and scoliosis (Fig. 38). Supporting orthoses may help the child to walk. Surgical treatment of deformities, particularly scoliosis, is sometimes needed.

Facioscapulohumeral muscular dystrophy. Usually autosomal dominant transmission. Becomes manifest in second decade with weakness and wasting of muscles around shoulders (Fig. 39), mouth and eyes. Life expectation is reasonable. Stabilization of the scapulae may improve function in the upper limbs.

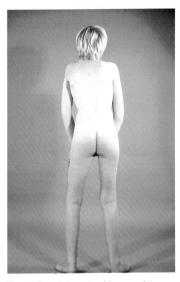

Fig. 37 Pseudohypertrophic muscular dystrophy.

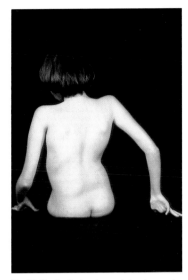

Fig. 38 Scoliosis due to weak trunk muscles in a congenital myopathy.

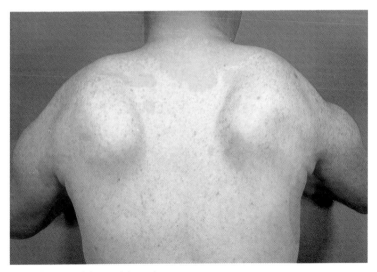

Fig. 39 Facioscapulohumeral dystrophy.

Spina bifida

Failure of closure of the vertebral canal during embryological development (Figs 40, 41). It is frequently associated with malformation of the spinal cord and nerve roots in the lumbar region.

Clinical features

These depend on the severity of the malformation. Tethering of nerve roots may cause only minor foot deformities but in severe forms there will be extensive paralysis, sensory loss in the lower limbs and loss of neurological control of pelvic viscera resulting in incontinence. Hydrocephalus is common in severe spina bifida because of blockage in the circulation of cerebrospinal fluid.

Orthopaedic aspects

Children with severe spina bifida who survive the neonatal period will often need correction of lower limb deformities and the provision of orthoses to allow walking. Gross spinal deformities can develop as the child grows.

Arthrogryposis multiplex congenita

A rare congenital condition of unknown cause in which the limb muscles show incomplete development.

Clinical features

Variable, depending on the extent of the disorder. The involvement is usually asymmetrical and the lower limbs are affected more than the upper. The limbs are thin, joints are stiff and often dislocated. Club foot deformity is common (Fig. 42).

Treatment

Deformities are usually difficult or impossible to correct surgically. Function is often better than might be expected.

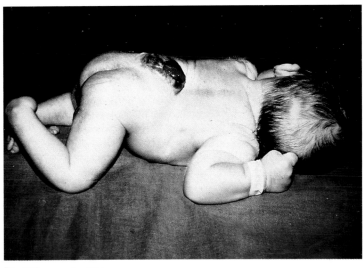

Fig. 40 Severe spina bifida.

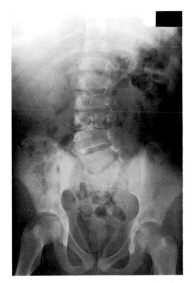

Fig. 41 X-ray of spina bifida. Note widening in lumbar region.

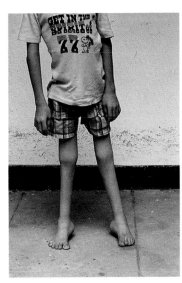

Fig. 42 Arthrogryposis.

Peroneal muscular atrophy

A not uncommon hereditary neuropathy, usually transmitted as an autosomal dominant trait.

Synonym   Charcot–Marie–Tooth disease.

Clincial features   Weakness and wasting of intrinsic muscles in the foot leading to pes cavus and clawing of toes (Fig. 43), usually manifest by 5–10 years. Weakness of calf muscles is common and hands and forearms may be involved. Ankle jerk reflex is often lost and there is diminution of vibration sense below the knee.

Treatment   See treatment of pes cavus (p. 133).

Neuropathic arthropathy

Destruction of a joint secondary to diminished pain sensation. Classically due to tabes dorsalis form of syphilis, but nowadays more often caused by diabetes mellitus or occasionally syringomyelia.

Synonym   Charcot's joint.

Clinical features   The joints in the lower limbs are more often affected in tabes and diabetes and those in the upper limb in syringomyelia.

 The condition often starts with acute swelling and discomfort. Later there is progressive destruction with deformity and instability of the involved joint but pain may be slight (Fig. 44).

Treatment   *Early.*   Rest and analgesics.

Late.   Stabilization by an orthosis when there is destruction and instability. Surgical arthrodesis is notoriously difficult to achieve and total joint replacements fail early.

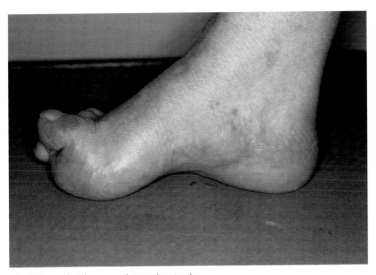

Fig. 43 Cavus foot in peroneal muscular atrophy.

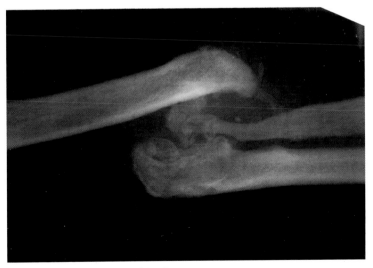

Fig. 44 Neuropathic destruction of the elbow.

4 / Skeletal dysplasias

A large group of congenital disorders which are characterized by generalized skeletal and often soft tissue abnormalities. Many, but not all, are heritable. Most are uncommon and some are extremely rare. Some of the more common and important disorders will be illustrated.

Osteogenesis imperfecta

Synonyms

Fragilitas ossium; 'brittle bone disease'.

Clinical features

There are several varieties but two main subtypes:

Congenita. Most severe form. Children may be born with fractures. Dwarfing and deformity are often severe in survivors. Sporadic or autosomal recessive pattern of inheritance.

Tarda. Most common form. Fractures are frequent in early childhood but their number becomes less as the child gets older. Autosomal dominant inheritance.

In both types there may be blue discoloration of the sclerae (Fig. 45), ligamentous laxity and poor wound healing.

X-ray examination shows slender bones (Fig. 46). Multiple fractures at different stages of healing may lead to confusion with a 'battered baby'. In severe cases repeated fractures lead to gross deformities of long bones (Fig. 47).

Treatment

Fractures usually heal with routine treatment. Severe bowing of long bones can be corrected by multiple osteotomies and stabilization with intramedullary rods, which are also used to prevent fractures.

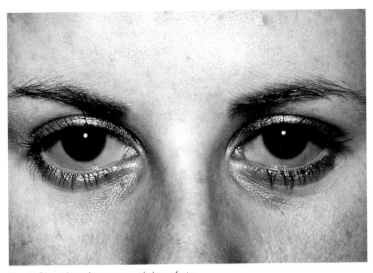

Fig. 45 Blue sclerae in osteogenesis imperfecta.

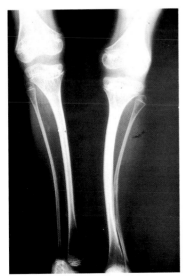

Fig. 46 Typical slender bones.

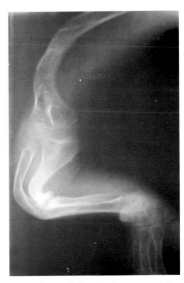

Fig. 47 Severe deformity due to repeated fractures.

Achondroplasia

A relatively common dysplasia in which the limbs are short but growth of the trunk is almost normal. Autosomal dominant inheritance.

Clinical features

Short limbs, short broad hands ('trident hands'), relative enlargement of the head, coarse facial features and lumbar lordosis (Fig. 48).

Treatment

Not usually needed. Limb lengthening is sometimes carried out. The lumbar spine is narrow in achondroplastic individuals and neurological complications due to spinal stenosis (p. 75) sometimes occur.

The mucopolysaccharidoses

A group of disorders characterized by abnormal storage of mucopolysaccharides due to the absence of enzymes necessary for their metabolism. Like all congenital disorders in which there is an enzyme deficiency, there is a recessive pattern of inheritance.

Clinical features

Often not manifest at birth. Later mental deficiency, dwarfing, hepatosplenomegaly and various skeletal deformities may appear. The clinical picture varies with the particular type of enzyme deficiency.

A protruding sternum (Fig. 49) is a striking feature of *mucopolysaccharidosis IV* (Morquio's disease, in which there is inability to metabolize keratan sulphate). Dwarfing is marked and the hands are stubby (Fig. 50).

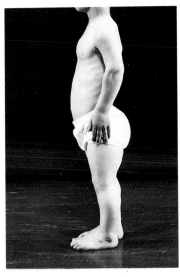

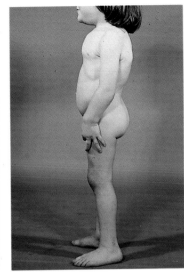

Fig. 48 Achondroplasia.

Fig. 49 Morquio's disease.

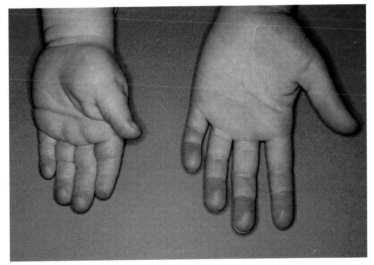

Fig. 50 The hand of a child with Morquio's disease next to that of a normal child of the same age.

Diaphyseal aclasis

A fairly common disorder, of autosomal dominant inheritance, in which exostoses form in the metaphyseal region of long bones.

Multiple exostoses.

Palpable bony lumps, typically around knees (Fig. 51), ankles and shoulders. The exostoses are bony outgrowths with cartilaginous caps and are therefore usually larger than they appear radiographically.

Extensive lesions may result in short stature and deformity of limbs. Malignant change occurs rarely.

Removal of unsightly exostoses or those causing pressure effects, e.g. on nerves. See also osteochondroma (p. 47).

Multiple enchondromatosis

A rare congenital disease, characterized by persistence of unmineralized cartilage within long bones. Sporadic in occurrence, with no genetic basis.

Dyschondroplasia; Ollier's disease.

Usually asymmetrical involvement. Hands are frequently affected by multiple cartilaginous 'tumours' or hamartomas (Figs 52, 53) which are often large and unsightly. Extensive lesions may cause shortening and deformity of limbs. Malignant change to a chondrosarcoma may occur.

Corrective osteotomy of deformed bones, or amputation of severely involved, functionally useless parts. See also enchondroma (p. 47) and chondrosarcoma (p. 53).

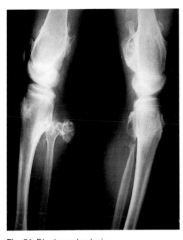

Fig. 51 Diaphyseal aclasis.

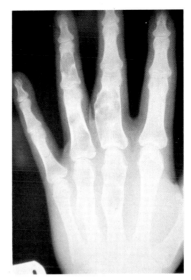

Fig. 52 Multiple enchondromatosis.

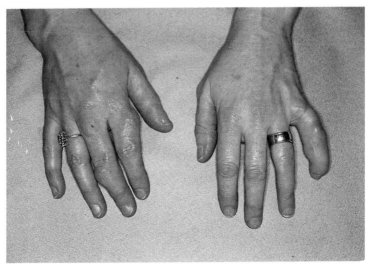

Fig. 53 Multiple enchondromatosis.

Multiple epiphyseal dysplasia

In this condition there is an abnormality of development of the epiphyses in many bones. There are probably several subtypes, but the most common variety is of autosomal dominant inheritance.

Clinical features

Usually apparent in childhood. Short stature and mild deformities are common (Fig. 54). Hands and feet are often short and stubby. The epiphyses are small, mottled and irregular. Typically the epiphyses of long bones in the lower limbs are worst affected and the appearance of the hips may be mistaken for Perthes' disease (p. 111). Osteoarthritis of involved joints, particularly the hips (Fig. 55), may occur at an early age.

Treatment

Medical and surgical management of osteoarthritis (pp. 7, 9).

Osteopetrosis

Abnormal remodelling of bone results in osteosclerosis, obliteration of marrow cavities and brittleness of bones. The condition is due to abnormal osteoclast function. Severe (congenita) and mild (tarda) forms are recognized, being autosomal recessive and dominant, respectively.

Clinical features

Congenita form is present at birth. In the tarda form, fractures occur in childhood. Osteopetrosis congenita has a poor prognosis. The infant often develops a severe anaemia due to obliteration of the marrow cavities. Radiographs show dense bones with abnormal modelling (Fig. 56).

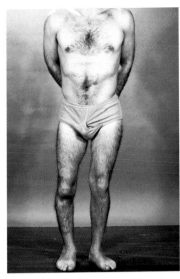

Fig. 54 Deformity in multiple epiphyseal dysplasia.

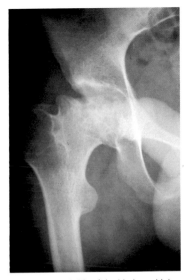

Fig. 55 Osteoarthritis of the hip in multiple epiphyseal dysplasia.

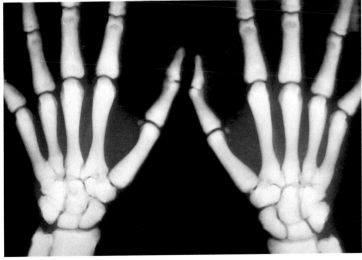

Fig. 56 Osteopetrosis.

Fibrous dysplasia

Replacement of areas of bone by fibrous tissue. The cause is unknown and the condition is not hereditary.

The lesions are usually found in the shafts and metaphyses of long bones. One bone (monostotic form) or several (polyostotic form) may be affected.

Clinical features

The lesions may be asymptomatic, or may present as local enlargement or deformity of the affected bone or bones (Fig. 57). Pathological fractures can occur and gross deformities may be produced if the disease is progressive. Polyostotic fibrous dysplasia is sometimes accompanied by extensive skin pigmentation and endocrine problems (Albright syndrome, Fig. 58).

Investigations

Radiographs show expansion of the bone with thinning of the cortex. The abnormal area may have a 'ground glass' appearance. Similar X-ray features are seen in hyperparathyroidism, which may be distinguished from fibrous dysplasia as there is biochemical evidence of abnormal calcium homeostasis.

In severe cases there will be radiological evidence of pathological fractures and deformities. A 'shepherd's crook' deformity of the hip (coxa vara) is typical (Fig. 59).

Treatment

Fractures are treated by standard methods. Corrective osteotomy of deformed bones may be needed.

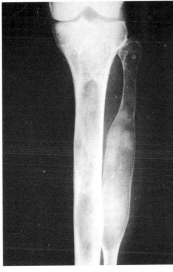

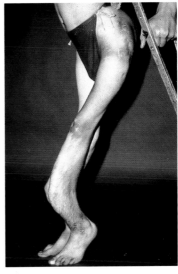

Fig. 57 Fibrous dysplasia affecting the tibia and fibula.

Fig. 58 Albright syndrome.

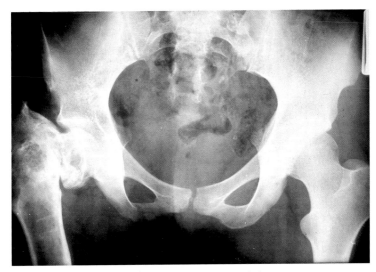

Fig. 59 Severe deformity of the right hip due to fibrous dysplasia.

Neurofibromatosis

A condition in which there is skin pigmentation, tumours of peripheral nerves, overgrowth of tissue and sometimes skeletal deformities. Inheritance is autosomal dominant.

Synonym

Von Recklinghausen's disease.

Clinical features

The manifestations are variable in extent and severity. 'Café au lait' skin patches (Fig. 60) and cutaneous fibromata and neurofibromata (Fig. 61) are the typical features.

Neurofibromata forming on peripheral nerves within the vertebral canal can compress the spinal cord. In severely affected individuals there may be local gigantism and a gross scoliosis (p. 67) can develop. Neurofibromata may undergo malignant change and this must be suspected if one enlarges rapidly.

Congenital pseudarthrosis of the tibia (Fig. 62) is a curious condition that is associated with neurofibromatosis. The tibia becomes progressively more deformed during childhood.

Treatment

Large, unsightly neurofibromata, or those causing local pressure effects, should be excised. Early spinal fusion is usually necessary if there is a progressive scoliosis.

Congenital pseudarthrosis of the tibia is notoriously difficult to treat; bone grafting and internal fixation procedures often fail to secure union.

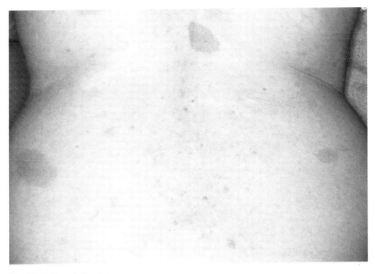

Fig. 60 'Café au lait' patches.

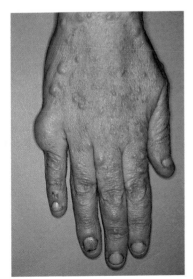

Fig. 61 Cutaneous neurofibromata.

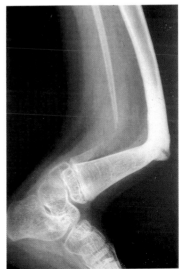

Fig. 62 Pseudarthrosis of the tibia.

Ehlers–Danlos syndrome

A syndrome characterized by joint and skin laxity and a haemorrhagic tendency. Mild forms are probably quite common but severe involvement (as seen in the 'india-rubber men' of side shows) is rare. Inheritance is autosomal dominant.

Synonym

Cutis laxa.

Clinical features

Joints are hyperextensible (Fig. 63). Recurrent dislocations of hips, patellae and shoulders are liable to occur. Scoliosis, kyphosis and foot deformities are not uncommon. The skin is lax and prone to heal poorly with 'tissue paper' scars especially over the knees (Fig. 64) and elbows.

Marfan syndrome

An uncommon condition characterized by abnormal height and long, thin extremities. Autosomal dominant inheritance.

Synonym

Arachnodactyly.

Clinical features

Manifestations are variable but the individual is usually tall with long slender fingers (Fig. 65) and toes. Generalized laxity of connective tissue may cause dislocation of the lenses of the eyes, aortic dilatation and incompetence. High arched palate and prognathism are common.

Orthopaedic aspects

Because of joint laxity, patients are prone to develop flat feet (p. 135), genu recurvatum, recurrent dislocation of the patellae (p. 123) and spinal deformities such as scoliosis (p. 67).

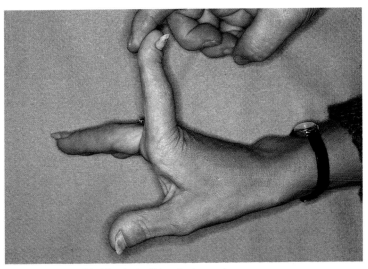

Fig. 63 Hyperextensible joints in the Ehlers–Danlos syndrome.

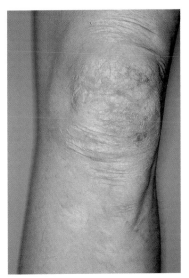

Fig. 64 'Tissue-paper' scars on the knee.

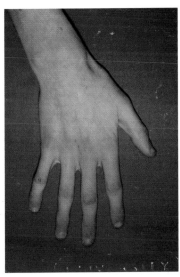

Fig. 65 The hand in Marfan syndrome.

Fibrous cortical defect

A common lesion which is usually an incidental X-ray finding in children aged 10–15. The femur is the most common site. The cause is unknown.

Radiographic appearance is characteristic. The lesion is eccentrically placed, initially in the metaphyseal region, but later moving away from the epiphyseal growth plate. Overlying cortex is thin or absent (Fig. 66).

Treatment

Not needed. Disappears in 2–5 years.

Solitary (unicameral) bone cyst

More common in boys. Usually found in proximal part of humerus or femur. May present in childhood as a pathological fracture (Fig. 67).

Treatment

Fractures usually heal but may recur. The cyst may disappear spontaneously. Healing is often hastened by injection of methylprednisolone acetate into the cyst.

Bone infarct/avascular necrosis

Death of bone follows loss of the local blood supply. Avascular necrosis is often idiopathic, but may be associated with alcoholism, steroid treatment or trauma. It is also seen in divers and tunnel workers ('caisson disease').

Clinical features

An infarct in the diaphysis of a long bone (Fig. 68) is often asymptomatic. If bone adjacent to a joint is affected there may be loss of support of articular cartilage and secondary osteoarthritis is common. This may require treatment (p. 7).

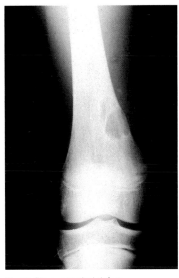

Fig. 66 Fibrous cortical defect.

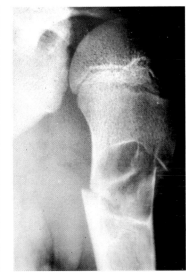

Fig. 67 Fracture through a solitary bone cyst.

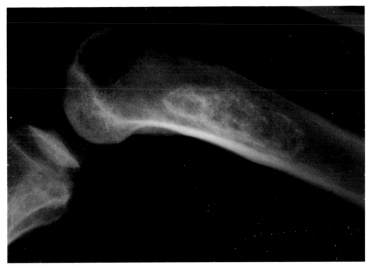

Fig. 68 Bone infarct in the medulla of the femur.

A variety of tumours occur in bone, ranging from the innocuous to the highly malignant. They require expert assessment and malignant tumours are best treated in specialist centres.

Diagnosis Depends on careful assessment of clinical, radiological and histological features. Atypical radiological features are common.

Osteochondroma

The most common benign bone tumour, often found near the knee (Fig. 69). It probably arises from the growth plate. It consists of a bony spur covered by a large cap of cartilage which is radiolucent (Fig. 70). If large and troublesome the lesion should be removed. See also diaphyseal aclasis (p. 35).

Chondroma

A benign cartilaginous tumour arising within bone (enchondroma) or from it (ecchondroma). It is common in the hand and may present as a pathological fracture (Fig. 71). Healing of the fracture is usually spontaneous, but curettage or bone grafting may be needed. See also multiple enchondromatosis (p. 35).

Osteoid osteoma

A small vascular tumour consisting of osteoid tissue within a nidus of sclerotic bone. It affects children and young adults, and common sites are the small bones of hands and feet, the neck of the femur, the tibia and spine. The tumour causes pain which is typically worse at night and relieved specifically by aspirin. Sclerotic bone may be seen on radiographs, and the lesion produces a striking 'hot spot' on an isotope bone scan (Fig. 72). Treatment is by complete excision.

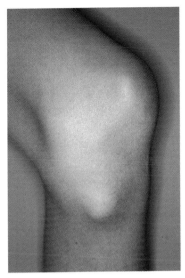

Fig. 69 An osteochondroma of the proximal tibia.

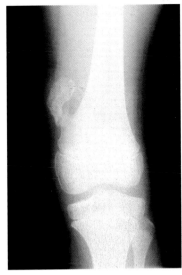

Fig. 70 Osteochondroma of femur.

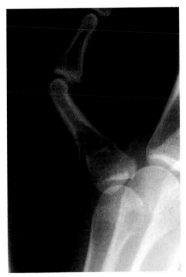

Fig. 71 An enchondroma in the proximal phalanx. Note the fracture.

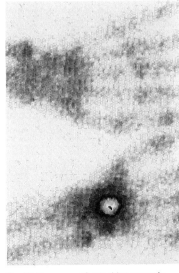

Fig. 72 Bone scan of osteoid osteoma in carpus.

Aneurysmal bone cyst

An expanded, blood-filled lesion typically found at the end of a long bone or in a vertebral pedicle. It may be caused by altered haemodynamics in bone rather than being a true neoplasm.

Clinical features

Most common in second and third decades of life. It causes pain and a swelling on the bone which may be pulsatile. Pathological fracture can occur.

Investigations

Radiographs show a cystic lesion. In long bones this lies in the metaphyseal region and does not encroach on the epiphysis (Fig. 73). Sometimes the cyst may 'explode' with loss of the overlying cortex.

Treatment

Drainage of the cyst and/or packing with bone chips. Radiotherapy is sometimes used if the lesion is surgically inaccessible.

Giant cell tumour

Tumours in which giant cells are seen on histological examination. The origin of these cells is not certain.

Synonym

Osteoclastoma.

Clinical features

Usually occurs in young adults. Common sites are the distal end radius (Fig. 74), distal end femur and proximal tibia. The lesion causes pain, swelling and occasionally pathological fracture.

Investigations

Radiographs show an expanded, localized lesion in the metaphysis, extending to the joint surface (Fig. 75).

Treatment

Excision if possible. The lesion may recur locally if excision is incomplete. Metastatic spread is rare.

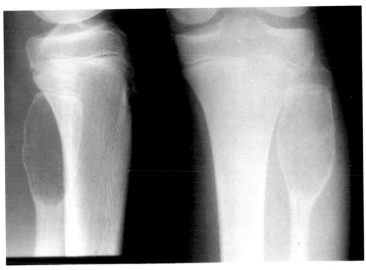

Fig. 73 Aneurysmal bone cyst in the fibula.

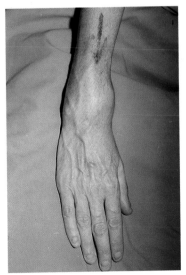

Fig. 74 Giant cell tumour in distal radius.

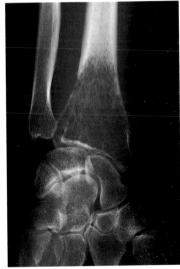

Fig. 75 Giant cell tumour in distal radius.

Osteosarcoma

A highly malignant tumour of bone-forming cells. Various histological subtypes are recognized.

Synonym

Osteogenic sarcoma.

Clinical features

A tumour of children and young adults but may occur in older people with Paget's disease of bone (p. 63). In young people the common sites are the proximal end of the tibia, the distal end of femur and the proximal end of humerus. The tumour causes pain, often worse at night, and swelling (Fig. 76). Pathological fractures can occur.

Investigations

Radiographs show destruction of cortical bone and sometimes new bone formation beneath raised periosteum (Codman's triangle, Figs 77, 78). Isotope bone scan shows increased uptake at the site of the lesion and any metastases. CT and MR scans will show any soft tissue extension. A biopsy is necessary for histological assessment, as with all bone tumours.

Treatment

Amputation well proximal to the tumour plus adjuvant chemotherapy has been the main treatment. However, limb-sparing surgery with local resection and reconstruction with a custom-built prothesis is preferable and is possible in many cases. Early metastasis to the lungs is common but survival has been improved by adjuvant chemotherapy. The parosteal type of osteosarcoma has a relatively good prognosis after adequate resection, but when osteosarcoma complicates Paget's disease (Fig. 79) the prognosis is extremely poor.

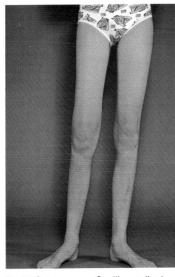

Fig. 76 Osteosarcoma. Swelling at distal end of right femur.

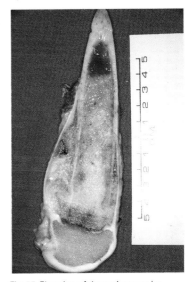

Fig. 77 Elevation of the periosteum by tumour.

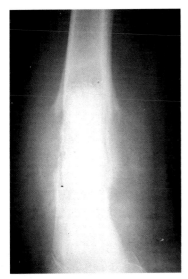

Fig. 78 Radiographic appearance of Codman's triangle.

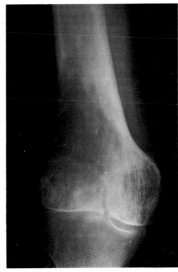

Fig. 79 Osteosarcoma in a femur affected by Paget's disease.

Chondrosarcoma

A malignant tumour derived from cartilage cells. It occasionally develops in enchondromata or osteochondromata, especially the multiple types (p. 35).

Clinical features

Usually occurs in middle-aged people. The tumour is slowly-growing and may become very large (Fig. 80).

Radiographs show either an expanding central lesion or a soft tissue shadow arising from the cortex of the bone. Calcification within the tumour is characteristic (Fig. 81).

Treatment

Because of slow growth and late metastasis there is a relatively good prognosis after amputation well proximal to the tumour.

Ewing's sarcoma

A malignant tumour of bone marrow. The precise cellular origin is uncertain.

Clinical features

Usually occurs in childhood. Typical sites are shaft of tibia, femur or humerus, or the pelvis (Fig. 82).

Radiographs may show an 'onion skin' appearance due to deposition of successive layers of subperiosteal bone. The periosteal reaction may cause confusion with osteomyelitis (p. 1), especially as the ESR is often raised and pyrexia may be present.

Treatment

Surgical resection if possible, with preceding chemotherapy. Otherwise treatment is by radical radiotherapy. Prognosis is variable but has been improved with chemotherapy.

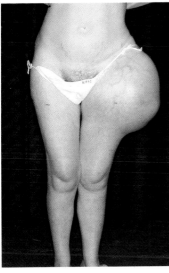

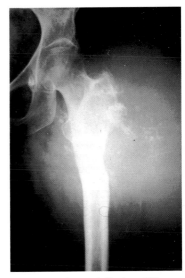

Fig. 80 Chondrosarcoma of proximal femur. A common site.

Fig. 81 X-ray shows calcification within tumour.

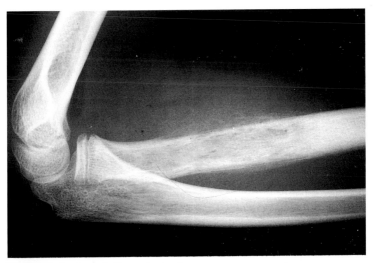

Fig. 82 Ewing's sarcoma in the proximal radius.

Multiple myeloma

Malignant tumour of plasma cells in marrow. It may initially be solitary but has usually progressed to multiple stage on presentation. Vertebrae, ribs, skull and pelvis are common sites.

Synonyms Plasmacytoma; myelomatosis.

Clinical features Bone pain, weakness, anaemia and weight loss. Investigations may reveal raised ESR, hypercalcaemia and abnormal proteins in serum and urine. Radiographs typically show vertebral collapse and sometimes 'pepper pot' lesions in the skull (Fig. 83).

Treatment Chemotherapy, and radiotherapy to local lesions. Prognosis is poor.

Metastatic bone tumours

Much more common than primary bone tumours. Primary tumours that commonly metastasize to bone occur in lung, breast, kidney and thyroid.

Clinical features Pain, swelling and pathological fractures (Fig. 84).

Treatment Isolated metastatic deposits warrant treatment to make the patient as comfortable as possible, even if the prognosis is poor. Internal stabilization of long bones should be carried out to prevent impending fractures from becoming complete. Internal fixation of complete fractures (Fig. 85) will relieve pain and minimize functional disability. Local radiotherapy may also be given. Pathological fractures often heal well.

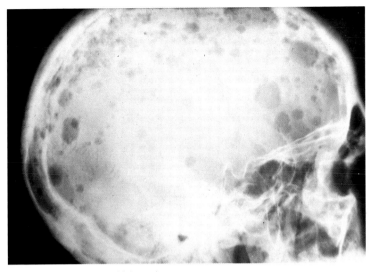

Fig. 83 Skull deposits in multiple myeloma.

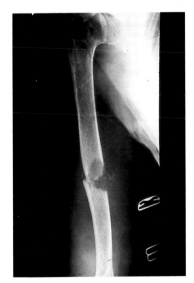

Fig. 84 Pathological fracture of the humerus due to metastatic tumour.

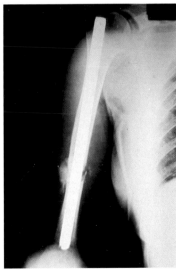

Fig. 85 Internal fixation of pathological fracture.

Synovial chondromatosis

An uncommon condition in which multiple cartilaginous foci form within synovial membranes. The foci may calcify and become detached to form loose bodies within the joint. These can cause mechanical derangement of the joint.

Clinical features

Affects the over 30 age group. Usually one joint is involved, most frequently the knee (Fig. 86). The joint swells and locks unpredictably when loose bodies (Fig. 87) are trapped between the joint surfaces.

Treatment

Removal of loose bodies and synovectomy.

Synovial sarcoma

A rare malignant soft tissue tumour. It is not now thought to arise from the synovium within joints but often occurs around joints and tendon sheaths.

Clinical features

Affects young adults. More common in the lower limb. Presents as a slowly growing, often painful, soft tissue swelling that may or may not be in the region of a joint (Fig. 88). A malignant soft tissue tumour must be suspected in these circumstances. The technique and approach for biopsy must be carefully considered to avoid compromising subsequent surgical treatment.

Imaging reveals a soft tissue mass which may contain calcific stippling (Fig. 89).

Treatment

Local excision is inadequate as the tumour invariably recurs. It is relatively resistant to chemo- and radiotherapy so radical excision of the tissue compartment containing the tumour or amputation is required. Metastasis to the lungs is common.

See also ganglion (p. 85) and villonodular synovitis (p. 105).

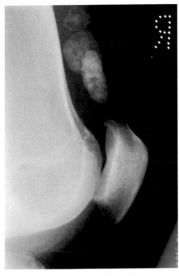

Fig. 86 Multiple loose bodies within the knee.

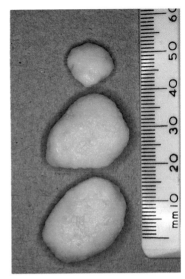

Fig. 87 The same after surgical removal.

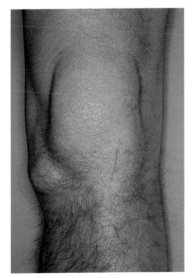

Fig. 88 Synovial sarcoma arising from medial aspect of the knee.

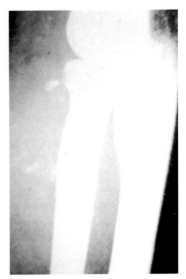

Fig. 89 Calcification within a synovial sarcoma of the forearm.

Osteoporosis

A generalized reduction in bone mass below the normal range for the particular age, sex and race of the individual. The bone is normal in quality but there is less of it than there should be.

Causes

Hormonal. Some bone loss is normal in the postmenopausal female, but if excessive it can lead to clinically apparent osteoporosis. Osteoporosis also occurs in thyrotoxicosis and Cushing syndrome.

Disuse. Immobilization, weightlessness in astronauts.

Others. Rheumatoid arthritis (p. 11), osteogenesis imperfecta (p. 31), Marfan syndrome (p. 43).

Clinical features

Often asymptomatic but fractures through weak bone are very common. Usual sites are wrist (Colles' fracture), neck of humerus, neck of femur (Fig. 90) and vertebrae. Back pain and loss of height result from multiple vertebral fractures (Fig. 91) which may also cause a dorsal kyphosis ('widow's hump', Fig. 92).

Investigations

Blood chemistry is usually normal. Osteoporosis is not radiologically apparent until more than 30% of the bone mass has been lost.

Treatment

Medical. There is no form of treatment that will reliably restore bone mass to normal.

Surgical. Treatment of patients with fractures due to osteoporosis accounts for a major part of the workload of most orthopaedic surgeons.

Prevention

Postmenopausal hormonal replacement therapy will prevent, but not replace, bone loss in susceptible women, but bone is lost rapidly if HRT is stopped.

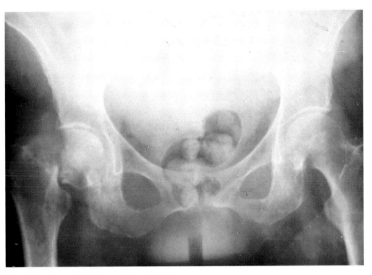

Fig. 90 A subcapital fracture of the right hip.

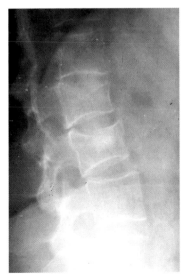

Fig. 91 Multiple vertebral fractures due to osteoporosis.

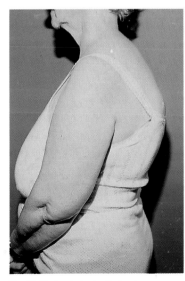

Fig. 92 Moderate kyphosis due to osteoporosis.

Rickets and osteomalacia

Osteomalacia and rickets are both due to inadequate intake or metabolism of vitamin D. Lack of vitamin D results in poor mineralization of the skeletal matrix. It may be due to inadequate diet, malabsorption or renal disease.

Rickets

The condition is caused by lack of vitamin D when skeletal growth is taking place.

Clinical features

Failure of mineralization of the rapidly growing metaphyseal region of bones (Fig. 93) leads to swelling of joints and bony deformities (Fig. 94). An associated myopathy can cause a waddling gait.

Investigations

Low serum calcium and phosphate, and raised alkaline phosphatase. Typical X-ray features (Fig. 93).

Treatment

Adequate replacement and maintenance dosage of vitamin D. Deformities of long bones may require corrective osteotomy.

Osteomalacia

The adult counterpart of rickets, usually affecting elderly people on a poor diet who may also have osteoporosis (p. 59).

Clinical features

Often unremarkable but may present with generalized skeletal pain, weakness and fractures through weakened bone.

Investigations

Blood picture similar to rickets. Radiographs may show pseudofractures (Looser's zones) in the pubic rami (Fig. 95) or other bones.

Treatment

Adequate replacement and maintenance dosage of vitamin D. Treatment of fractures.

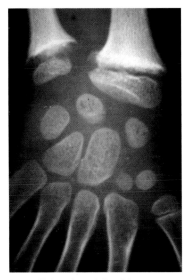

Fig. 93 Rickets. Irregularity of the metaphyses of the radius and ulna.

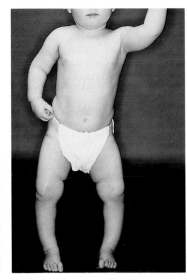

Fig. 94 Bow legs caused by rickets.

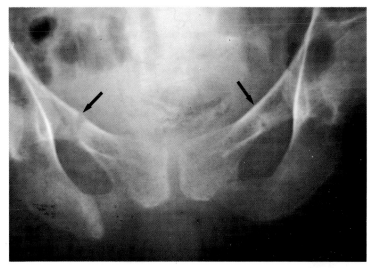

Fig. 95 Osteomalacia. Pseudofractures in the pubic rami.

Paget's disease of bone

Although loosely classed as a metabolic bone disease, Paget's disease of bone is a disorder of unknown aetiology in which there is thickening and deformity of one or several bones. The rates of formation and resorption of bone appear to be uncoordinated.

Synonym

Osteitis deformans.

Clinical features

Affects men more than women. Rare below the age of 40 but increasingly common with age. Pelvis, femur, tibia, skull and vertebrae are common sites.

The disease is asymptomatic in the majority but may cause pain, swelling and deformity of affected bones (Fig. 96). Thickening of the calvarium results in increase of head size and change of its shape (Fig. 97).

Investigations

Plasma alkaline phosphatase raised and urinary hydroxyproline excretion increased.

Localized osteoporosis is an early radiographic feature. Later there is coarse trabeculation and loss of distinction between the cortex and medulla. Microfractures may occur on the convex border of long bones (Fig. 98).

Complications

Microfractures may progress to complete fractures (Fig. 99). Compression of nerves by affected bones may cause deafness or paraplegia. Osteoarthritis can occur when bone adjacent to a joint is affected. Osteosarcomatous change is uncommon but must be suspected if there is an increase in local pain; the prognosis is poor.

Treatment

Medical. Analgesics, calcitonin, diphosphonates.

Surgical. Internal fixation of fractures is sometimes necessary.

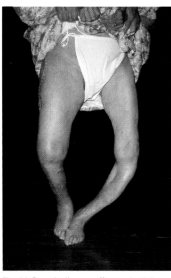

Fig. 96 Paget's disease affecting both legs.

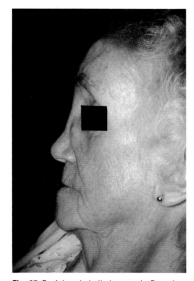

Fig. 97 Facial and skull changes in Paget's disease.

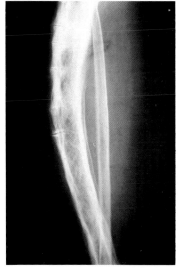

Fig. 98 Typical microfractures in the tibia.

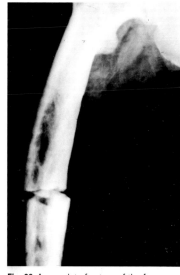

Fig. 99 A complete fracture of the femur.

Torticollis

Tilting and rotation of the head.

Types

Infantile. Due to idiopathic contracture of one of the sternomastoid muscles (Fig. 100). It usually develops during infancy. A swelling in the sternomastoid muscle may be noted before the contracture occurs.

Treatment is by stretching the muscle or surgical division.

Secondary. Secondary to imbalance of extrinsic eye muscles, cervical lymphadenopathy or acute muscle spasm.

Treatment is by correcting the underlying abnormality.

Spasmodic. A type of 'tic' or dystonia in which there is sudden uncontrollable writhing of the neck. The cause is unknown.

No form of surgical or medical treatment has been found to be particularly effective, although botulinus toxin may be helpful.

Cervical rib

An abnormal bony or fibrous development of the costal process of the 7th cervical vertebra (Fig. 101).

Clinical features

Symptoms are frequently absent and the rib may be an incidental finding. Occasionally, vascular or neurological symptoms may occur which can be attributed to pressure on the subclavian artery or lower trunks of the brachial plexus by the rib or, more commonly, a fibrous band attached to it. Young adults are usually affected.

Treatment

Mild symptoms respond to physiotherapy. Surgical removal of the rib or band is indicated only if there are objective, worsening neurological or vascular signs.

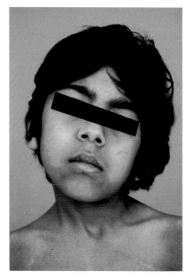

Fig. 100 Infantile torticollis.

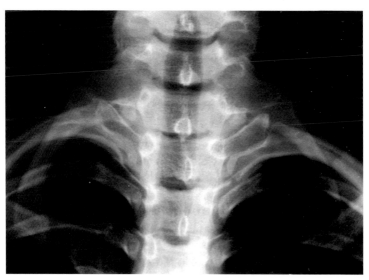

Fig. 101 Bilateral cervical ribs.

Scoliosis

Lateral curvature of the spine.

Postural. A compensatory scoliosis will occur when one leg is shorter than the other. The spine is structurally normal and a postural curve will not become fixed.

Structural. The curve is due to an abnormality in the spine.
   The two types can be distinguished by asking the patient to lean forwards (Fig. 102), when a postural scoliosis will disappear.
   Most structural curves are idiopathic in origin but some are due to neuromuscular dysfunction (e.g. in poliomyelitis and muscular dystrophies) or congenital bony abnormalities in the spine (Fig. 103). Scoliosis is also a feature of many skeletal disorders (e.g. Marfan syndrome, neurofibromatosis).

Depending on the cause, the curve may commence at any age in the growing child. Any part of the thoracolumbar spine may be involved. Untreated structural scoliosis gets worse during growth in most cases. In addition to deformity, an untreated patient may develop cardiorespiratory problems if the thoracic spine is affected. Radiographs confirm the extent of the deformity (Fig. 104).

Young children must be treated in a brace to prevent increasing deformity. Older children are treated by surgical fusion of the affected spinal segment. Residual deformity can often be improved by the use of implants such as Luque rods that are attached to posterior elements of the vertebrae.

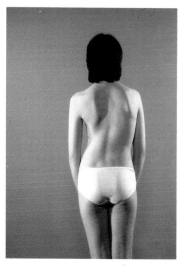
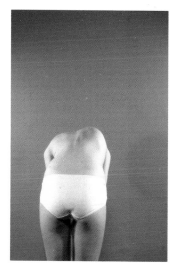

Fig. 102 A structural scoliosis remains when the patient leans forward.

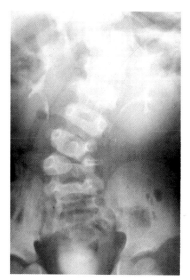

Fig. 103 Congenital vertebral anomalies.

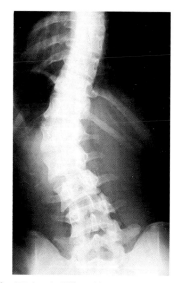

Fig. 104 A typical idiopathic scoliosis.

Discitis

An uncommon condition of unknown cause in which there is narrowing and sometimes calcification of the intervertebral disc space.

Clinical features

Affects children aged 6–14. The lumbar spine is usually involved. The child complains of pain in the back or abdomen, and may be pyrexial. Examination reveals muscle spasm and limitation of spinal movement. Radiological narrowing of the disc space (Fig. 105) may take a week or two to appear.

Treatment

Bedrest until symptoms settle.

Vertebra plana

Collapse of a vertebral body, probably caused by an eosinophilic granuloma of bone. Uncommon.

Synonym

Calvé's disease.

Clinical features

Affects children aged 2–12. There is local discomfort, usually in the thoracic spine. X-ray examination shows collapse of a vertebral body with preservation of the disc spaces (Fig. 106).

Treatment

Rest until pain settles. Bone may reform.

Adolescent kyphosis

A common condition in which there is abnormal development of the ring epiphyses of the thoracic vertebral bodies.

Synonym

Scheuermann's disease.

Clinical features

Produces a round-shouldered deformity in 12–16 age group (Fig. 107). There may be mild discomfort. X-rays show wedging of vertebral bodies (Fig. 108).

Treatment

Seldom needed but in more severe cases a brace may be needed to prevent increasing kyphosis.

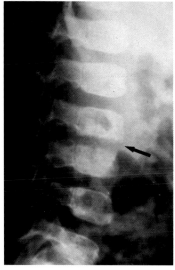

Fig. 105 Irregular disc space in discitis.

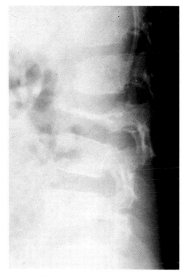

Fig. 106 Vertebra plana.

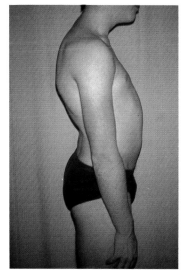

Fig. 107 Adolescent kyphosis.

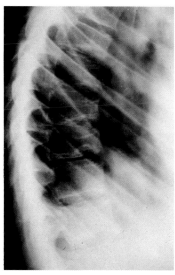

Fig. 108 Wedging of vertebra in adolescent kyphosis.

Spondylolysis

A defect in the pars interarticularis of a vertebra, usually in the lower lumbar region (Fig. 109).

Clinical features

May predipose to low back pain in adult life but is frequently an incidental finding in adults who do not have back pain.

Treatment

Symptoms, if any, are relieved by wearing a spinal support.

Spondylolisthesis

A defect or elongation of the pars interarticularis associated with forward slipping of one vertebra relative to another or the sacrum (Fig. 111). It is often due to a congenital or developmental abnormality of the vertebra.

Clinical features

Can be a cause of low back pain in childhood. A step between the spinous processes may be palpable. Occasionally an acute slip occurs and the youngster presents with a stiff spine, increasing lumbar lordosis and spasm of the hamstring muscles, causing the knees to be held in slight flexion (Fig. 110).

Spondylolisthesis in adults is usually due to degenerative changes in the interfacetal joints of the vertebra but may be caused by injury or pathological fractures.

Treatment

Surgical fusion of the appropriate spinal segments is usually indicated for symptomatic spondylolisthesis in young people.

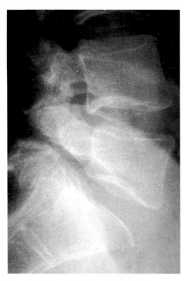

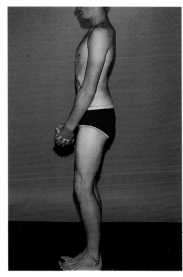

Fig. 109 Spondylolysis with defect in pars interarticularis of L5.

Fig. 110 Acute spondylolisthesis: the typical posture.

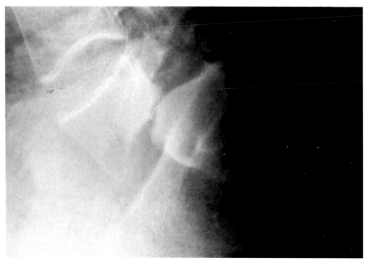

Fig. 111 Spondylolisthesis between L5 and S1.

Prolapsed intervertebral disc

A rupture of the gelatinous nucleus pulposus of the intervertebral disc through the annulus fibrosus, usually in a posterolateral direction.

Synonym

'Slipped disc'.

Clinical features

Often happens spontaneously but may follow acute strain when lifting. The lumbar spine is the usual site. The extruded disc material produces pressure on a nerve root. Pressure on the L5 or S1 nerve roots causes pain down the back of the leg (sciatica), often made worse by coughing. Normal lumbar lordosis is lost (Fig. 112) and spinal movements are restricted. To relieve pressure on the nerve the spine is tilted to one side (Fig. 113); the direction of tilt depends on the position of the prolapse in relation to the nerve root. Passive flexion of the hip with the leg held straight is limited (straight leg raising test) and pressing on the tibial nerve in the popliteal fossa will cause pain. There may be motor and sensory impairment with loss of tendon jerks, the neurological pattern depending on the root involved. Rarely a central disc prolapse will cause pressure on the cauda equina and urinary symptoms; this is a surgical emergency.

Investigations

Magnetic resonance imaging will show indentation of the dura at the level of the disc prolapse (Figs 114, 115).

Treatment

Most will settle with bedrest, analgesia and spinal support. Surgical removal of the disc prolapse is considered only if sciatica or neurological symptoms fail to resolve with adequate conservative treatment, or if there is a central disc prolapse with cauda equina symptoms.

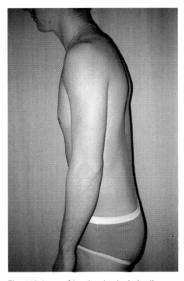

Fig. 112 Loss of lumbar lordosis in disc prolapse.

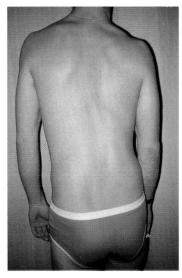

Fig. 113 Muscle spasm and lumbar spinal tilt.

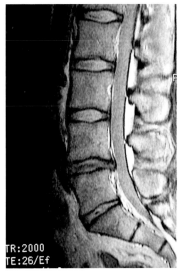

Fig. 114 MR scan showing L4/5 disc prolapse.

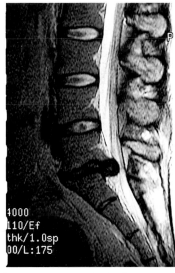

Fig. 115 MR scan showing L5/S1 prolapse.

Osteoarthritis

For a general description of osteoarthritis, see page 7. Degenerative osteoarthritis of the spine is extremely common. The clinical symptoms often bear little relationship to the severity of radiological changes.

Types

There are several clinical forms:

Cervical spondylosis (Fig. 116). OA of the cervical spine may cause pain in the neck and arms by entrapment of nerve roots in the intervertebral foramina. The symptoms usually ease with time. In the acute phase, treatment is by warmth, neck support and analgesics. Neck traction is sometimes helpful.

Lumbar spondylosis (Fig. 117). Degenerative changes in the intervertebral joints of the lumbar spine. The condition may be an incidental X-ray finding. Acute episodes of pain and stiffness are treated symptomatically.

Spinal stenosis. Narrowing of the vertebral canal by osteophytes arising from the interfacetal joints. Pressure on the cauda equina can cause claudication-like symptoms with a normal peripheral circulation. Myelography shows obstruction to free movement of the radio-opaque medium (Fig. 118). Decompression of the vertebral canal by laminectomy may be necessary if symptoms are severe.

Ankylosing vertebral hyperostosis (Forestier's disease). Large bony outgrowths arising from the anterior part of the vertebrae at multiple levels, often in the thoracic region (Fig. 119). Stiffness and discomfort are often slight and are treated symptomatically.

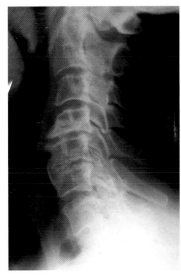

Fig. 116 Cervical spondylosis.

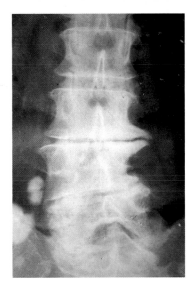

Fig. 117 Lumbar spondylosis.

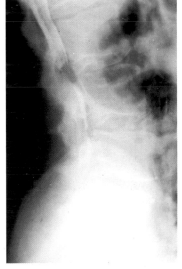

Fig. 118 Spinal stenosis.

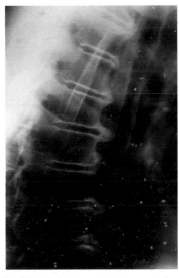

Fig. 119 Ankylosing vertebral hyperostosis.

Congenital high scapula

The scapula develops in the embryo opposite the 4th, 5th and 6th cervical vertebrae and migrates to its usual thoracic position between the 9th and 12th weeks of intrauterine life. When failure of descent of one scapula occurs there is an ugly asymmetry in the line of the shoulders (Fig. 120) and limitation of movements, especially abduction.

Synonym Sprengel's shoulder.

Cause The cause is unknown but there is often an abnormal band of fibrous tissue, cartilage or bone connecting the superior angle of the scapula to the cervical spine. Associated congenital anomalies are common.

Treatment Function of the shoulder is often good, but both appearance and function can be improved by early surgical correction.

Frozen shoulder

Loss of glenohumeral movement that may be secondary to injury, minor inflammatory conditions, immobilization of the arm, or of idiopathic origin.

Synonym Adhesive capsulitis.

Clinical features Usually unilateral. The middle-aged are most often affected. Night pain is a prominent feature. There is loss of both active (Fig. 121) and passive glenohumeral movements.

Treatment Anti-inflammatory analgesics. Physiotherapy is contraindicated in the early active phase. The condition is self-limiting but may take up to 2 years to resolve.

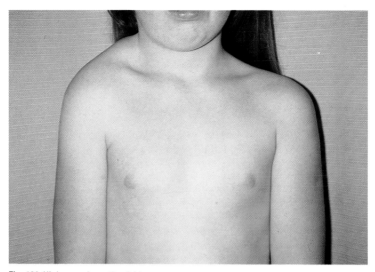

Fig. 120 High scapula on the right.

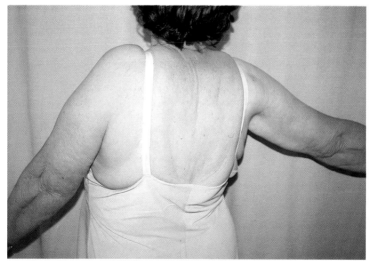

Fig. 121 Frozen left shoulder. Loss of active glenohumeral movement.

Rupture of long head of biceps

Usually a spontaneous rupture occurring without significant stress. Probably caused by degenerative changes in the tendon.

Clinical features

Most common in middle-aged men. Patient may feel that 'something has given way' around the shoulder but pain and functional disability are slight.

The muscle belly displaces distally and looks abnormal when the elbow is fixed against resistance (Fig. 122).

Treatment

Reassurance and normal use.

Acute calcific tendonitis

A not uncommon condition in which periarticular inflammation is associated with the formation of a deposit of calcium salts. The shoulder is the joint that is most often affected and the cause is unknown.

Clinical features

Affects 30–50 age group most often. The pain is acute in onset and very severe. The joint may be hot and tender. Discomfort settles rapidly over a few days but the condition can recur or affect the other shoulder. Radiographs show the typical calcium deposit (Fig. 123) although this may not be visible early in the attack.

Treatment

Strong analgesics and anti-inflammatory drugs. Aspiration or surgical removal of the calcific deposit will shorten the attack.

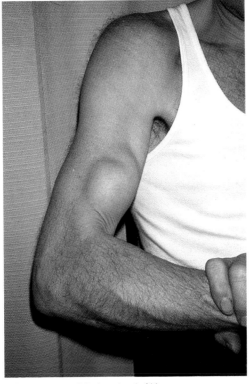

Fig. 122 Rupture of the long head of biceps.

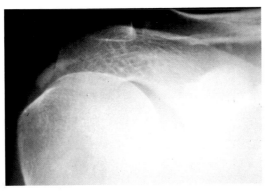

Fig. 123 Acute calcific tendonitis.

Tear of rotator cuff

Acute rupture of the supraspinatus tendon is usually due to age-related changes in the tendon.

Clinical features

Most common in elderly men. After a minor injury or strain there is inability to abduct the shoulder actively. Passive abduction is full (compare with frozen shoulder, p. 77).

X-ray examination is negative, but in cases of long standing the head of the humerus migrates proximally to impinge on the acromion (Fig. 124).

Treatment

Early surgical repair in active patients. In the very elderly the tendon is degenerate and difficult to repair; conservative treatment to keep the shoulder mobile is preferable.

Winging of scapula

The scapula is stabilized by the serratus anterior muscle which is innervated by the long thoracic nerve (C5, 6, 7). Damage to the nerve in its long course may result in paralysis of the muscle and winging of the scapula (Fig. 125). In many cases there is no history of trauma and it is thought that the nerve is damaged by a viral mononeuritis.

Clinical features

Young men are most often affected and the right shoulder more than the left. Winging is noted about 2 weeks after an acute attack of pain in the shoulder. In the similar condition of *neuralgic amyotrophy* there may be more extensive paralysis and wasting of muscles around the shoulder.

Treatment

Spontaneous recovery is usual but may take up to 2 years.

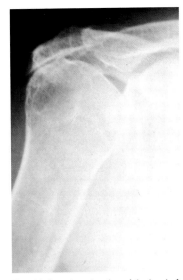

Fig. 124 Superior migration of the head of the humerus after a tear of the rotator cuff.

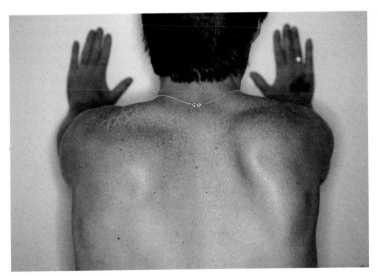

Fig. 125 Winging of the right scapula.

Tennis elbow

Discomfort over the lateral epicondyle of the humerus (Fig. 126). It is very common. The less common medial epicondylitis ('golfer's elbow') is a similar condition.

Synonym Lateral epicondylitis.

Cause May develop after an acute strain but usually arises without significant trauma. The pathology is obscure but tearing or degeneration of tendinous tissue in the extensor origin has been postulated.

Clinical features Tenderness over the lateral epicondyle with increased pain when the fingers are extended against resistance. Tenderness over the extensor muscle mass may be found when the posterior interosseous nerve is compressed in the supinator muscle—'atypical tennis elbow'.

Treatment The condition is self-limiting but can recur. Symptomatic treatment by local steroid injection, ultrasound and a tennis elbow strap may be helpful. Surgical release may be required for posterior interosseous nerve entrapment.

Olecranon bursitis

Inflammatory swelling of the bursa over the olecranon. It may be infective or traumatic in origin.

Clinical features The swelling is obvious (Fig. 127). It is soft and attached to underlying bone.

Treatment *Infected.* Antibiotics. Surgical drainage may be needed.

Traumatic. Local steroid injection may speed resolution.
  Excision of the bursa is avoided if possible as healing of the overlying skin may be slow.

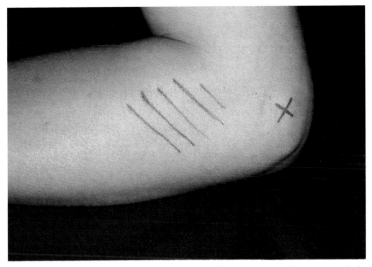

Fig. 126 The site of pain in tennis elbow is marked with a cross. Pain is felt in the hatched area when there is entrapment of the posterior interosseous nerve.

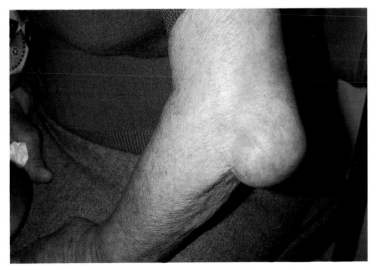

Fig. 127 Olecranon bursitis.

De Quervain's tenosynovitis

Thickening of the fibrous sheath of the first dorsal compartment of the wrist which contains the tendons of extensor pollicis brevis and abductor pollicis longus.

Cause

Uncertain, but repetitive movements may aggravate the condition.

Clinical features

Most common in middle-aged women. There is pain and swelling proximal to the radial styloid process. Discomfort is aggravated by passive ulnar deviation of the wrist, especially when the thumb is gripped (Finkelstein's test, Fig. 128).

Treatment

Conservative. Rest in cast. Injection of cortisone into compartment (*not* tendon).

Surgical. Release of tendon sheath. Any subcompartments must be released. Damage to the terminal branches of the radial nerve must be avoided or a troublesome neuroma may form.

Ganglion

A cystic swelling associated with joints or synovial tendon sheaths. It consists of a fibrous swelling containing viscous fluid. The pathogenesis is obscure but may be due to herniation of synovial tissue or connective tissue breakdown.

Clinical features

Most commonly seen on the dorsoradial aspect of the wrist in young adults (Fig. 129). It sometimes causes discomfort, but is often asymptomatic.

Treatment

About 50% disappear spontaneously. Aspiration or excision is indicated if the ganglion is large or symptomatic, but recurrence is common.

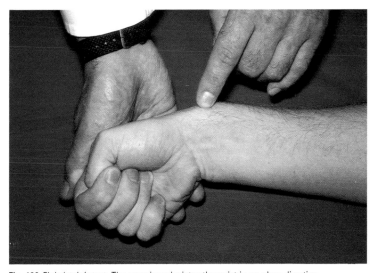

Fig. 128 Finkelstein's test. The examiner deviates the wrist in an ulnar direction.

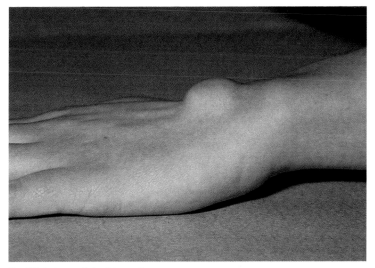

Fig. 129 A dorsoradial wrist ganglion.

Kienböck's disease

Sclerosis and collapse of the bone (Fig. 130).

Synonyms   Avascular necrosis of lunate bone; lunatomalacia.

Cause   Unknown. It may be due to traumatic damage to the blood supply. Relative shortening of the ulna is often noted but the significance is uncertain.

Clinical features   Affects young adults. Usually there is diffuse wrist pain but the condition may be asymptomatic.

Treatment   *Early.*   Rest in plaster and correction of discrepancy in lengths of radius and ulna.

Later stages.   Intercarpal arthrodesis, and wrist arthrodesis if there is secondary osteoarthritis.

Madelung's deformity

An uncommon congenital deformity of the wrist in which there is increased dorsal and radial bowing of the distal end of the radius, with an exaggerated radial and volar tilt of the distal articular surface.

Cause   Unknown. It is a typical feature of dyschondrosteosis, a skeletal dysplasia. Some cases are post-traumatic and others are idiopathic.

Clinical features   Usually bilateral. It may cause pain in the wrist. The deformity is obvious both clinically and radiologically (Fig. 131).

Treatment   Surgical correction is rarely required.

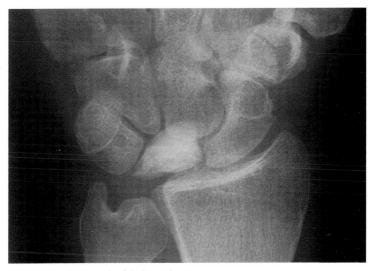

Fig. 130 Avascular necrosis of the lunate bone.

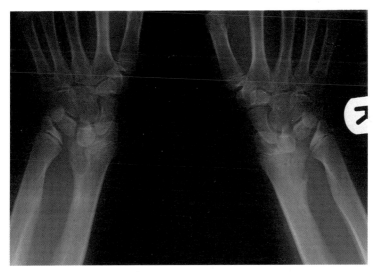

Fig. 131 Bilateral Madelung's deformities.

Congenital anomalies

Classification

- Failure of formation
- Failure of differentiation
- Duplication
- Undergrowth
- Overgrowth
- Constriction band anomalies
- Associated with skeletal dysplasias
- Miscellaneous.

A few representative examples will be illustrated.

Causes

There may be a clear pattern of inheritance or there may a non-heritable extrinsic cause (e.g. the effect of thalidomide), but in many cases no cause is identified. The hand deformity may be isolated or associated with other congenital anomalies.

Treatment

May not be necessary and should be directed to improving function rather than cosmesis. Major reconstructive procedures should be completed before school age if possible.

Failure of formation

May be transverse or longitudinal.

A common level for a transverse defect is the upper third of the forearm (Fig. 132). The deformity is not inherited, and treatment is by early fitting of a prosthesis.

In longitudinal defects there is often absence or hypoplasia of a digit (Fig. 133). Failure of formation of the radius produces the 'radial club hand' deformity (Figs 134, 135). It is sporadic in occurrence and was one of the typical deformities caused by taking thalidomide in early pregnancy. ➡

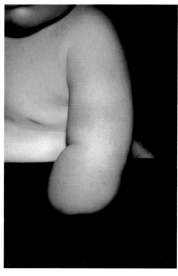

Fig. 132 Congenital absence of the forearm.

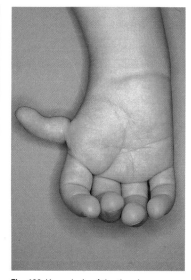

Fig. 133 Hypoplasia of the thumb.

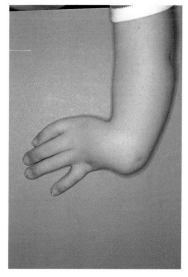

Fig. 134 Radial club hand.

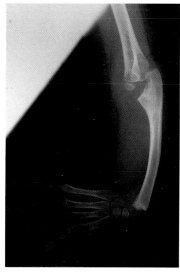

Fig. 135 Radial club hand (X-ray).

Failure of differentiation

A typical example would be syndactyly—failure of separation of the digits (Fig. 136). It may be an isolated anomaly or associated with other malformations. The inheritance is variable.

In simple syndactyly the fingers are joined by skin alone. Surgical separation produces a good cosmetic and functional result.

In complex syndactyly the fingers are joined by soft tissues and bone. Surgical separation is difficult but worthwhile.

Duplication

The possession of extra digits (polydactyly) is a fairly common example (Fig. 137). Inheritance is variable. An obviously abnormal and functionless digit should be removed.

Associated with skeletal dysplasias

The hand may be oddly shaped in achondroplasia (p. 33), the mucopolysaccharidoses (p. 33), multiple epiphyseal dysplasia (p. 37) and Marfan syndrome (p. 43). Function is good, however, and treatment is not needed.

Miscellaneous

Many hand deformities cannot be classified easily into one of the groups. A typical example is the condition of camptodactyly, a congenital flexion deformity of the proximal interphalangeal joints most often seen in the little fingers (Fig. 138). It is usually of autosomal dominant inheritance. Function is satisfactory and treatment is rarely needed.

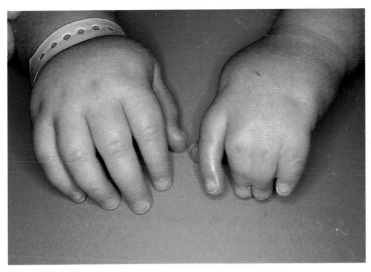

Fig. 136 Syndactyly.

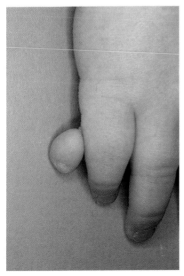

Fig. 137 Polydactyly.

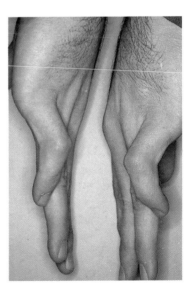

Fig. 138 Camptodactyly.

Trigger finger

A common condition in which the finger or thumb cannot be actively straightened from the flexed position.

Synonyms

Stenosing tenosynovitis; locking finger.

Cause

This is unknown, although the condition is more common in diabetics and patients with rheumatoid arthritis, who may have flexor tenosynovitis (p. 11). Sometimes a nodule forms on the tendon which can be withdrawn from the tendon sheath by the action of the powerful flexor muscles but tends to stick in the mouth of the sheath when the hand relaxes, thus preventing full extension of the digit.

Clinical features

Most common in the middle-aged, although a congenital flexion deformity of the thumb due to the same mechanism is sometimes seen in infants and young children (Fig. 139).

The onset is usually spontaneous. Patients complain of 'sticking' or 'locking' of a finger or thumb which has to be straightened passively (Fig. 140). Pain on straightening the digit may be referred to the proximal interphalangeal joint.

Treatment

Injection of hydrocortisone into the fibrous flexor sheath around the tendon.

Surgical release of the mouth of the sheath if injection fails.

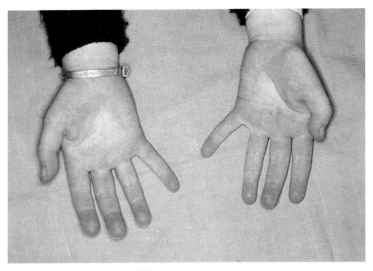

Fig. 139 Left trigger thumb in a child.

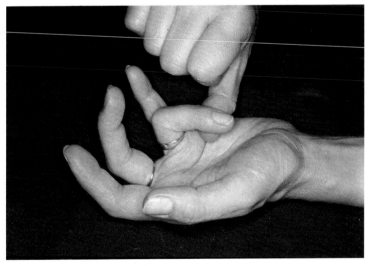

Fig. 140 Straightening a trigger digit.

Dupuytren's disease

A common condition in which the palmar and digital fascia becomes thickened and sometimes contracted.

Cause

Unknown. It is common in people of North European descent but very rare in other races. There is a strong hereditary element, the trait appearing to be transmitted as an autosomal dominant with variable penetrance.

Patients often attribute the condition to previous injury or heavy manual work but it is just as common in people with sedentary jobs.

Pathology

Aggregates of contractile fibroblasts form within the fibrous palmar and digital fascia.

Clinical features

Usually occurs in middle and old age. The ulnar side of the hand is most often affected.

The earliest stage is thickening and nodularity of the palmar fascia without contracture (Fig. 141). Knuckle pads (Garrod's pads, Fig. 142) are sometimes seen at an early stage of the disease on the dorsum of the proximal interphalangeal joints, although they can occur in the absence of other signs of Dupuytren's disease.

In some patients the nodules form bands of fibrous tissue that pass into the digits. These bands can undergo contraction with resultant flexion deformities of the affected digits (Fig. 143). Secondary contractures of the capsules of the proximal interphalangeal joints may occur.

Treatment

Depends on the severity and extent of the disease. Mild Dupuytren's disease does not require treatment. Surgery is indicated for early progressive contracture and established deformity. The operation of choice is removal of the abnormal fascia (local fasciectomy) which should be done before secondary joint contractures have become established. Recurrence and extension of the disease after operation is not uncommon.

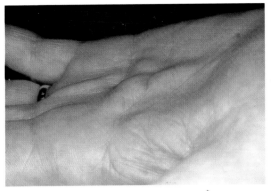

Fig. 141 Dupuytren's tissue in the palm of the hand.

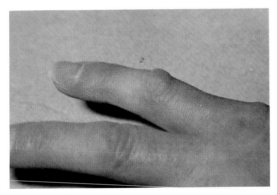

Fig. 142 Knuckle pad on little finger.

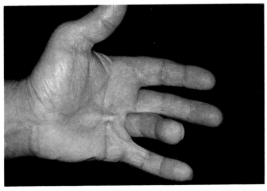

Fig. 143 Typical contracture affecting the ring finger.

Nerve lesions

The hand is supplied by the median, ulnar and radial nerves.

Nerves may be divided in any open injury of the hand or forearm. Surgical repair should be performed by an expert under ideal conditions if maximum function is to be restored. Full recovery is not always achieved in mixed motor and sensory nerves in adults, but useful function is regained in many cases.

Median nerve

Motor: to abductor pollicis brevis, opponens pollicis, part or all of flexor pollicis brevis and the radial two lumbrical muscles in the hand. In the forearm it supplies all the flexor muscles with the exception of flexor carpi ulnaris and the ulnar half of flexor digitorum profundus.

Sensory: to skin over the thenar eminence, palmar surface of the thumb and the radial two and one half fingers.

Variations in the motor and sensory distributions are not uncommon.

Clinical conditions

Loss of function in the median nerve results in inability to abduct and oppose the thumb (Fig. 144). In longstanding cases there is wasting of the thenar muscles (Fig. 145). When the median nerve is damaged proximally in the arm there is loss of active flexion of the index finger and thumb. The other fingers can be flexed by the action of the ulnar innervated portion of flexor digitorum profundus. This produces the characteristic 'sign of benediction' on attempting to make a fist (Fig. 146). See also carpal tunnel syndrome (p. 99). ➡

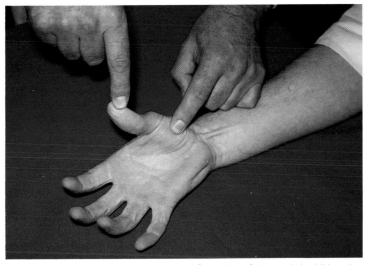

Fig. 144 Testing normal abduction of the thumb. Contraction of the muscle is visible and palpable.

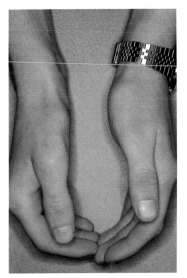

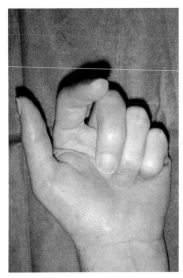

Fig. 145 Wasting of the thenar muscles in the right hand.

Fig. 146 Proximal median nerve lesion.

Ulnar nerve

Motor: to the intrinsic muscles of the hand that are not supplied by the median nerve.

Sensory: to the palmar aspect of the ulnar one and a half fingers and the whole of the back of the hand except for the area supplied by the radial nerve.

Clinical conditions

Damage to the ulnar nerve leads to wasting of the intrinsic muscles, most obviously the first dorsal interosseous. The little and ring fingers adopt a position of slight flexion with hyperextension at the metacarpophalangeal joints—the 'ulnar claw hand' (Fig. 147). Clawing is more marked when the ulnar nerve is damaged at the wrist than when it is damaged more proximally, because of imbalance between the intrinsic and extrinsic muscles acting on the fingers.

Froment's sign. When the patient attempts to grip a flat object between the thumb and the hand the flexor pollicis muscle (innervated by the median nerve) comes into action because the adductor pollicis is paralysed; hence the thumb on the affected side flexes at the interphalangeal joint (Fig. 148).

Loss of function in the ulnar nerve is not as disabling as loss of the median nerve. There is some loss of dexterity and weakness of grip but function of the hand is often surprisingly good.

Radial nerve

The radial nerve supplies sensation to the dorsoradial surface of the hand. Loss of this sensation is seldom disabling. It is motor to the extrinsic extensors of the fingers and wrist; proximal damage to the nerve causes wrist drop.

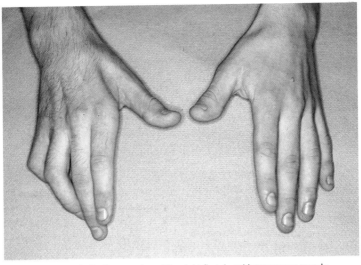

Fig. 147 Ulnar paralysis. Note wasting of the right first dorsal interosseous muscle.

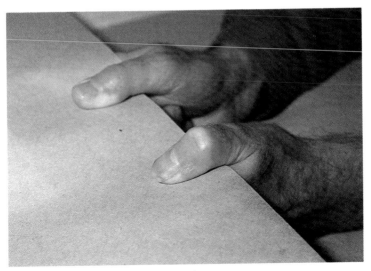

Fig. 148 Positive Froment's sign in the left hand.

Carpal tunnel syndrome

A common condition in which there is compression of the median nerve beneath the flexor retinaculum at the wrist.

Cause

Usually idiopathic but may be caused by any condition that decreases the space in the carpal tunnel, e.g. rheumatoid arthritis (proliferating synovium), pregnancy and hypothyroidism (fluid retention), abnormal muscle bellies and ganglia.

Clinical features

The patient, who is typically a middle-aged woman, is woken during the night with burning or bursting discomfort in the hand. Discomfort is not always confined to the median nerve distribution; often the whole hand and forearm are affected.

Relief is obtained by some activity such as shaking the hand, running cold water over it, or getting up and making tea. The hand may feel heavy and numb in the morning.

Examination often shows no abnormality. Only in advanced cases is median nerve paresis (p. 97) detectable clinically. Unforced flexion of the wrist for about one minute reproduces the symptoms in about 75% of patients (Phalen's test, Fig. 149).

Treatment

Conservative. Splinting the wrist will often give symptomatic relief. Diuretics and cortisone injection beneath the carpal tunnel may also be effective.

Surgical. Division of the flexor retinaculum. A visible constriction in the median nerve (Fig. 150) is not always found.

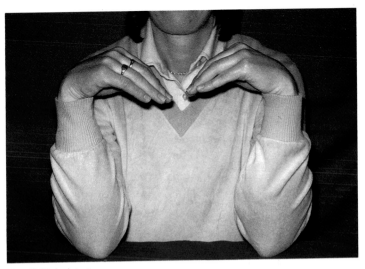

Fig. 149 Phalen's test.

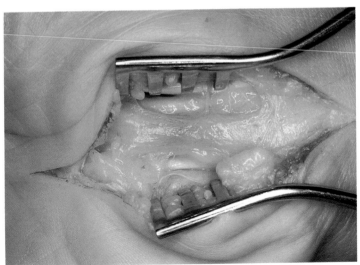

Fig. 150 Constriction of the median nerve seen at surgical decompression.

Osteoarthritis

For a general description of OA, see page 7. Although OA typically affects large weight bearing joints such as the hip or knee, it is not uncommon in the hand.

Clinical features

Older women are most often affected. Typically the distal interphalangeal joints are involved, showing the classic Heberden's nodes which are due to osteophytes around the joints (Figs 151, 152). A 'mucous cyst' (p. 105) may develop.

OA often affects the trapeziometacarpal joint at the base of the thumb (Fig. 153). The patient has pain on gripping, for example when wringing out clothes. An adduction contracture of the thumb is not uncommon (Fig. 154).

Treatment

OA of the distal interphalangeal joints seldom requires surgical treatment.

Trapeziometacarpal OA may cause disabling pain in everyday activities. Surgical treatment by excision or replacement arthroplasty may be necessary if it does not respond to conservative treatment by rest and anti-inflammatory analgesics.

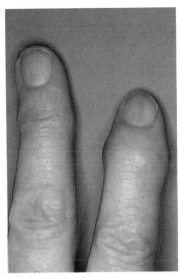

Fig. 151 Heberden's nodes in index finger.

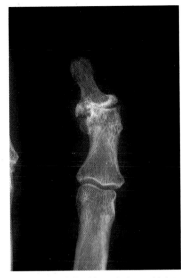

Fig. 152 OA of distal interphalangeal joint.

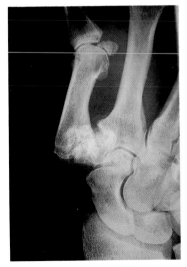

Fig. 153 Trapeziometacarpal OA.

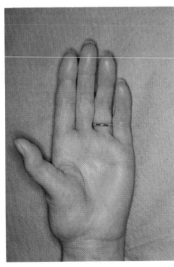

Fig. 154 Typical thumb deformity in trapeziometacarpal OA.

Common swellings

Ganglion

For a general description of ganglions, see page 85. The most common site for a ganglion is on the dorsum of the wrist, but they also occur on the volar aspect.

A fibrous flexor sheath ganglion presents as a firm swelling at the base of the finger (Fig. 155) which may cause discomfort on gripping handles or steering-wheels.

A 'mucous cyst' is a ganglion arising from a terminal interphalangeal joint affected by osteoarthritis (p. 103) (Fig. 156).

Pigmented villonodular synovitis

A lobular tumour, probably of synovial origin, arising from joints and tendon sheaths. It often has a yellowish appearance on section because it contains lipid and haemosiderin. Giant cells are not always present.

Synonym

Giant cell tumour of tendon sheath.

Clinical features

Most common in middle age. The tumour presents as a firm, painless swelling on the flexor aspect of the finger or the dorsal aspect of the distal joint (Fig. 157).

Treatment

Excision. It may recur if excision is incomplete.

Implantation dermoid

A subcutaneous cyst caused by growth of skin cells which have been implanted by a penetrating injury. Almost invariably found on the flexor aspect of the hand (Fig. 158).

Treatment

Excision.

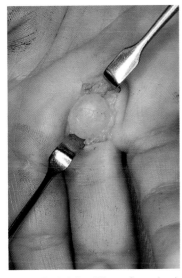

Fig. 155 Typical site of fibrous flexor sheath ganglion.

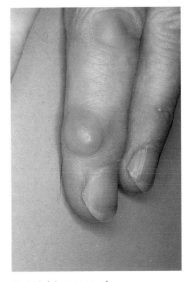

Fig. 156 A 'mucous cyst'.

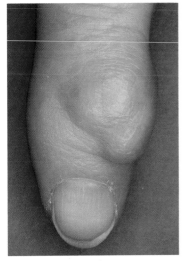

Fig. 157 Pigmented villonodular synovitis.

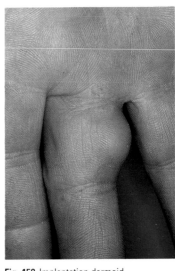

Fig. 158 Implantation dermoid.

Congenital dislocation of the hip (CDH)

Occurs in about 3–5/1000 newborn children in Britain but the incidence varies considerably between different countries and races. For example, it is almost unknown in the Bantu. The condition may be unilateral or bilateral.

Cause

Unknown. It is more common in females, first-born children and after breech delivery. There may be a family history.

Clinical features

Early. All newborn children should be screened for CDH. The flexed hips are abducted; if a hip is dislocated it will usually slip back into the acetabulum with a palpable 'clunk' during this manoeuvre (Ortolani's test, Fig. 159). The examination should be done when the child is relaxed after a feed.

Radiographic confirmation of the clinical diagnosis is difficult because the hips are largely cartilaginous at this stage, but ultrasonography may be helpful.

Late. Unless detected in the neonatal period the diagnosis is seldom made before the child begins to walk, when a limp and leg length discrepancy will become apparent. Radiographs will then confirm the diagnosis (Fig. 160).

Treatment

Early. A device such as the Pavlik harness is used to maintain the hip in flexion and abduction. The head will usually relocate in this position. For best results, treatment should begin in the neonatal period and be maintained until the hip is stable.

Late. Treatment becomes considerably more difficult as the child becomes older. Open reduction and surgical reorientation of the acetabulum and femoral head are usually necessary. Early degenerative osteoarthritis is liable to occur unless the hip is completely congruent.

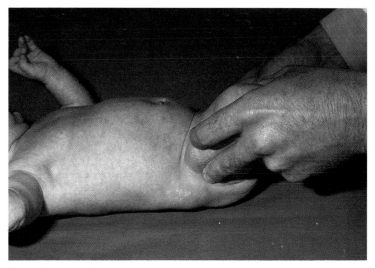

Fig. 159 Testing for CDH.

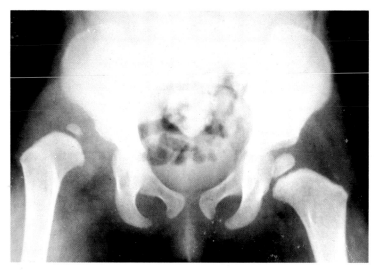

Fig. 160 Untreated CDH in a child.

Femoral anteversion

The angle of anteversion lies between the axis of the head and neck of the femur and the plane of the front of the femoral condyles. There is a wide variation in this angle in children. If the angle is greater than normal the range of internal rotation at the hips will be increased (Fig. 161) and the range of external rotation correspondingly diminished.

Clinical features

Children with marked femoral anteversion walk with their feet and patellae turned inwards (Fig. 162). This intoeing or 'hen-toed' gait is a cause of parental concern. When sitting the child favours the 'W' position (Fig. 163); this is probably a result rather than a cause of the anteversion.

Treatment

This is not required. Spontaneous improvement almost always occurs by the age of 10 without any treatment. There is seldom any disability in children in whom full correction does not occur. The condition should be regarded as a variation of normal development, rather than a pathological disorder, and the parents reassured.

Intoeing gait due to femoral anteversion should be distinguished from intoeing due to metatarsus adductus (p. 133). Intoeing may also be caused by mild genu valgum ('knock-knees') since in this condition the feet are turned inwards to provide a stable base for walking.

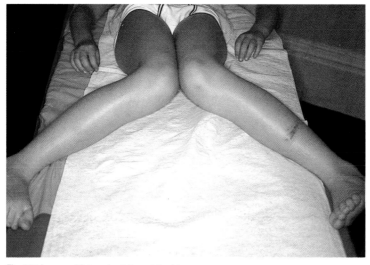

Fig. 161 Increased internal rotation at the hips.

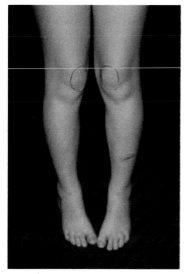

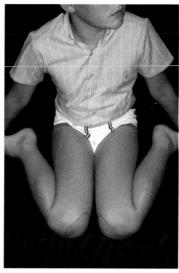

Fig. 162 Intoeing due to femoral anteversion.

Fig. 163 The 'W' position.

Perthes' disease

An idiopathic collapse of the ossific centre in the head of the femur.

Synonym

Coxa plana.

Cause

Unknown but thought to be due to a disturbance in blood supply to the head of the femur.

Clinical features

Affects children aged 4–10. The child may be noted to limp or complain of pain in the groin or the inner aspect of the knee.

On examination of the hip in the acute phase there is usually limitation of active and passive movement. Muscle spasm is often visible on passive rotation of the extended hip (Fig. 164).

Investigations

Radiographs show collapse and fragmentation of the ossific centre (Fig. 165).

Progress

Recovery takes up to 2 years and is variable. Some children show full recovery without active treatment whereas others have a progressive deformity of the femoral head and develop osteoarthritis in early adult life. Some idea of the prognosis can be gained from the extent of changes in the head of the femur on initial radiographs.

Treatment

Traction while there is muscle spasm. Weight bearing should be avoided until hip movements are full.

Pelvic or femoral osteotomy may be indicated in some children to prevent progressive deformity of the femoral head, but the results are unpredictable.

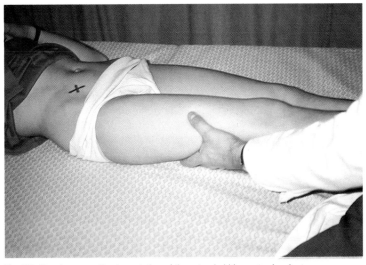

Fig. 164 Muscle spasm. Passive rotation of the extended hip causes involuntary contraction of the abdominal muscles.

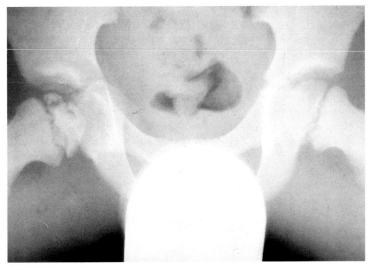

Fig. 165 Perthes' disease affecting the right hip.

Slipped upper femoral epiphysis

A posteroinferior displacement of the proximal femoral epiphysis, occurring in the absence of major injury.

Synonym

Adolescent coxa vara.

Cause

Unknown, but 50% of children affected have an abnormality of body build, either obesity or extreme slenderness. A hormonal effect on the growth plate may be involved.

Clinical features

Occurs in 10–18 age group. Both hips are affected in 25%. The displacement happens gradually but may be accelerated by falls at sports or games. There is a limp, with pain in the hip or referred to the knee.

On examination there is limitation of abduction and internal rotation of the hip. In severe slips, the whole leg will be externally rotated.

Investigations

An early slip is easily missed on AP films of the hip (Fig. 166) but is much more clearly seen on lateral films taken with the hips in the 'frog' position; these should always be done (Fig. 167). A complete slip is unmistakable (Fig. 168).

Treatment

Early slip. The epiphysis should be stabilized as a matter of urgency, using fine pins passed up the neck of the femur.

Severe slip. Manipulative reduction is avoided because of the risk of causing avascular necrosis of the head of the femur. The deformity must be corrected by open reduction or upper femoral osteotomy.

Complications

Deformity, avascular necrosis, loss of articular cartilage (chondrolysis), secondary osteoarthritis.

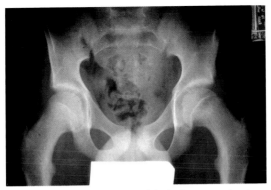

Fig. 166 Early slip of left femoral epiphysis. Anteroposterior view.

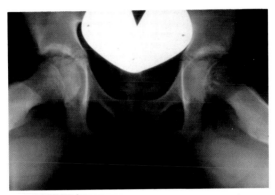

Fig. 167 Early slip of left femoral epiphysis. 'Frog lateral' view with hips flexed and abducted.

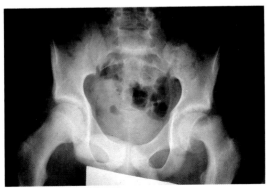

Fig. 168 Severe slip of left femoral epiphysis.

Osteoarthritis

For a general description of OA, see page 7. OA of the hip is a common and disabling condition of middle-aged and elderly people.

Causes

It may be primary (idiopathic) or secondary to previous injury, Perthes' disease (p. 111), slipped upper femoral epiphysis (p. 113), avascular necrosis (p. 45) and congenital subluxation (partial dislocation) of the hip (p. 107).

Clinical features

Pain, stiffness, loss of movement, deformity and a limp. The most common deformity is a combined flexion, adduction and external rotation contracture of the hip which causes an apparent leg length discrepancy. A flexion deformity can be demonstrated by flexing the good hip until the normal lumbar lordosis is eliminated (Thomas' test, Fig. 169).

Investigations

Radiographs show loss of joint space, sclerosis of periarticular bone, osteophytes and cysts (Fig. 170).

Treatment

Mild disability. Analgesics, physiotherapy, use of a stick (in hand opposite affected hip) and weight loss if appropriate.

Severe disability. Hip replacement is by far the most common treatment in the elderly but because of the risk of long-term complications (p. 9) it should be avoided in younger people if possible. Upper femoral osteotomy can be performed at any age if the range of hip movement is good, but the results are unpredictable. In young people arthrodesis is still the most suitable operation, although it is fortunately rarely necessary.

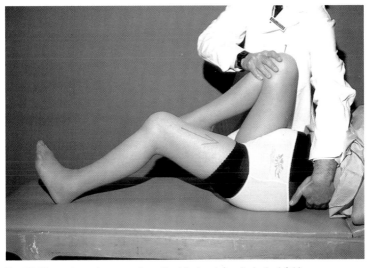

Fig. 169 Thomas' test, demonstrating a fixed flexion deformity in the left hip.

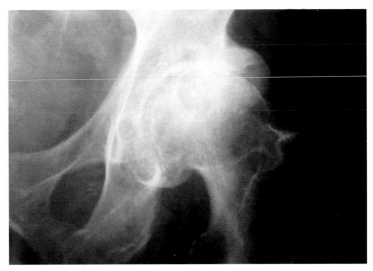

Fig. 170 Osteoarthritis of the hip.

Bursitis

Enlargement of bursae around the knee is a common complaint.

Cause

Usually secondary to chronic irritation (e.g. kneeling) but may occasionally be due to infection.

Clinical features

A firm, transilluminable swelling in the location of one of the bursae. The semimembranous bursa is often affected in childhood. In adults the prepatellar and infrapatellar bursae (Fig. 171) are more often enlarged.

Treatment

Irritative bursitis usually settles without treatment if the cause is avoided. Infected bursae may require surgical drainage and antibiotic treatment.

Baker's cyst

A synovial herniation into the popliteal fossa (Fig. 172).

Cause

Usually secondary to some intra-articular problem such as osteoarthritis (p. 127) or a degenerative meniscus, particularly if the underlying problem is associated with a chronic synovial effusion.

Clinical features

A swelling which varies in size in the popliteal fossa. Occasionally the cyst ruptures and synovial fluid tracks into the calf muscles, mimicking a deep venous thrombosis.

Treatment

Excision of the cyst is seldom indicated unless the underlying condition can be treated, as otherwise recurrence is almost always the rule.

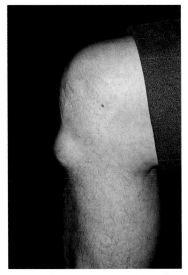

Fig. 171 Infrapatellar bursa.

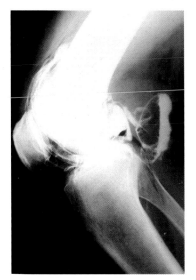

Fig. 172 Arthrogram showing a Baker's cyst.

Disorders of the menisci

Acute tears

Clinical features

Commonly caused by twisting injuries and therefore often seen in young, fit people who play a lot of sport. The medial meniscus is damaged more often than the lateral. It may tear to form a tag or a longitudinal split (a 'bucket handle'). The torn part of the meniscus can displace between the femoral and tibial condyles, causing sudden inability to extend the knee ('locking'). Recurrent effusions are common.

Investigations

Inspection of the knee through an arthroscope (Fig. 173) will usually confirm the diagnosis.

Treatment

Partial or complete removal of the affected meniscus. Meniscectomy by arthroscopic techniques is now preferred to open operation.

Degenerative tears

Clinical features

Common in the middle-aged and elderly. May cause aching discomfort and sometimes an effusion. Locking is not a symptom as the tear lies horizontally within the meniscus and displacement does not occur.

Treatment

Symptoms often settle spontaneously. Meniscectomy should be avoided if possible as it may accelerate degenerative change in articular cartilage.

Meniscal cysts

Clinical features

May be associated with degenerative changes within a meniscus, most often the lateral one. There is a tense swelling on the joint line and aching discomfort.

Treatment

Excision of the cyst plus meniscectomy if the meniscus is clearly abnormal, otherwise the cyst may recur (Fig. 174).

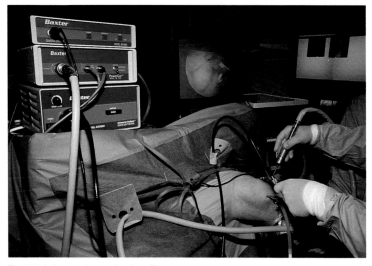

Fig. 173 Arthroscopic examination of knee.

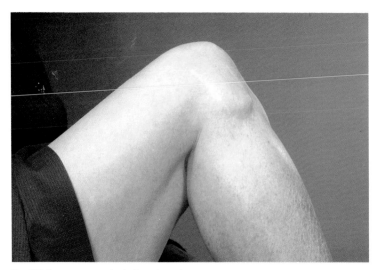

Fig. 174 A recurrent cyst in the lateral meniscus.

Tibial apophysitis

Synonym

Osgood–Schlatter's disease.

Clinical features

Common in boys aged 12–14 years. There is pain over the tibial tuberosity which is palpably and visibly enlarged (Fig. 175). Discomfort is often aggravated by activity. Radiographs show fragmentation of the epiphysis (Fig. 176).

Treatment

The condition is self-limiting and the long-term function of the knee is normal. There is no specific treatment, but if the knee is painful on strenuous exercise it is sensible to restrict athletic pursuits. Very occasionally a small separate ossicle may remain after the tibial apophysis has fused and may warrant excision.

Ossification in the medial collateral ligament

A condition that occurs sometimes after injury to the proximal attachment of the medial collateral ligament on the femoral condyle.

Synonym

Pellegrini–Stieda's disease.

Clinical features

Local swelling and discomfort. Radiographs confirm the diagnosis (Fig. 177).

Treatment

Local anaesthetic and corticosteroid injection.
   A similar clinical picture is seen in acute calcific tendonitis (p. 79) around the knee, but the onset is usually more acute and there is no history of previous injury. The treatment is the same.

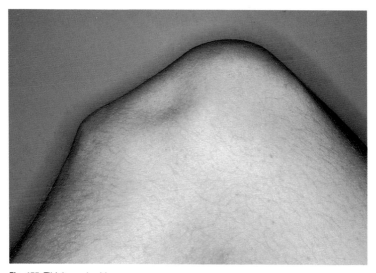

Fig. 175 Tibial apophysitis.

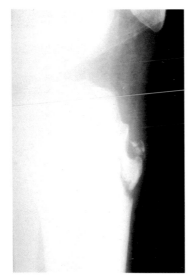

Fig. 176 Tibial apophysitis.

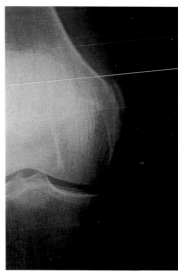

Fig. 177 Calcification in the medial collateral ligament.

Anterior knee pain

Retropatellar knee pain is extremely common in teenaged girls. It is occasionally attributable to changes in the articular cartilage of the patellae ('chondromalacia patellae', Fig. 178), although most often no cause is found.

Clinical features

Discomfort, often worse on stairs. Clinical examination is often negative, although there may be joint laxity and moderate genu valgum. Radiographs are normal. Arthroscopy will reveal any changes in the articular cartilage, if present.

Treatment

Mild analgesics such as soluble aspirin. Restriction of activities may be necessary for a while but should be kept to a minimum. Various operations have been described for chondromalacia patellae but the results are unpredictable and frequently disappointing.

Recurrent subluxation of the patella

Clinical features

Most common in teenaged girls and young women. Subluxation occurs in a lateral direction and the knee gives way suddenly, causing the patient to fall to the ground.

On examination there may be mild joint laxity, genu valgum and often a small, high patella. The patient is apprehensive when the patella is pushed laterally.

Tangential radiographs usually show hypoplasia of the lateral femoral condyle and incongruity of the patellofemoral articulation (Fig. 179).

Treatment

Physiotherapy to develop the quadriceps muscle. Surgical realignment of the patella if symptoms persist.

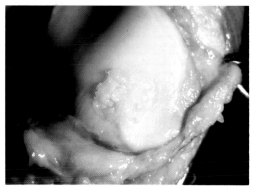

Fig. 178 Chondromalacia patellae.

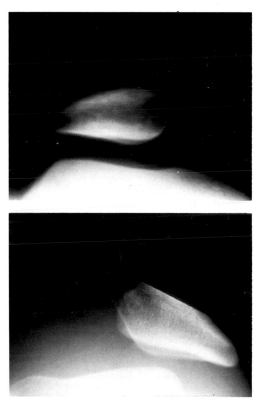

Fig. 179 Subluxation of the patella. The other knee is shown above for comparison.

Osteochondritis dissecans

In this condition there is separation of an avascular fragment of bone and cartilage from the surface of the joint. The medial femoral condyle of the knee is most often affected (Fig. 180), but it can occur in other joints.

Clinical features

Usually affects boys aged 10–18. The initial complaint is local discomfort but if the fragment separates it may become trapped between the joint surfaces, causing sudden locking (Fig. 181). Secondary osteoarthritis can occur in early adult life if the joint is badly affected.

Treatment

Before separation. The fragment may heal back in place with rest. Drilling the bone may encourage revascularization.

After separation. The fragment should be pinned back in place if possible and not simply removed.

Blount's disease

An uncommon condition in which there is abnormal growth of the medial part of the proximal tibial epiphysis. The cause is unknown; similar deformities can occur after injury or infection.

Synonym

Tibia vara.

Clinical features

West Indian children are most often affected.

Infantile type. Accentuation of the normal bow-legged appearance of the toddler, progressing to severe deformity in later childhood. The varus deformity is associated with an internal rotational deformity of the tibia.

Adolescent type. Unilateral. Onset is at age 8–15 (Fig. 182). Final deformity not as severe as infantile type.

Treatment

Correction by osteotomy.

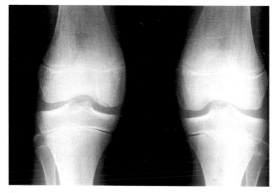

Fig. 180 Early osteochondritis dissecans, right medial femoral condyle.

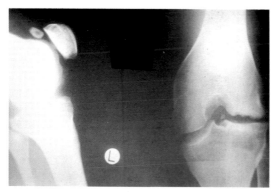

Fig. 181 Irregularity of joint surfaces and a loose body.

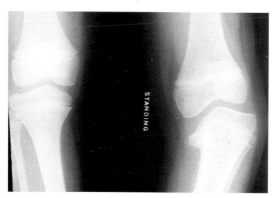

Fig. 182 Blount's disease, left tibia.

Osteoarthritis

For a general description of osteoarthritis, see page 7. Osteoarthritis of the knee is very common. It is usually secondary to some recognizable cause such as obesity, previous injury or previous meniscectomy (Fig. 183).

Clinical features

Often bilateral. The main complaints are of stiffness and pain. On examination there is often a flexion contracture, or genu varum if only the medial compartment of the knee is affected (Fig. 184).

Investigations

Radiographs show the usual features of OA affecting one or more of the articular areas of the knee.

Treatment

Conservative. Analgesics, walking aids, weight loss if appropriate.

Surgical. Indicated if symptoms are not controlled by conservative measures. Realignment of the tibia by upper tibial osteotomy (Fig. 12) is often helpful if OA is confined to the medial compartment and there is a varus deformity (Fig. 185). Arthrodesis of the knee is seldom indicated. Although it is successful in relieving pain, the inability to bend the knee is a serious inconvenience. Total knee replacement is used if there are extensive osteoarthritic changes. Knee replacement is not as successful as hip replacement in patients with OA as they are often overweight and physically active. As a result, early loosening of the prosthetic joint can be a serious problem.

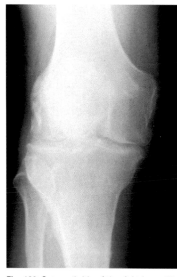

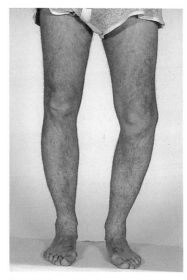

Fig. 183 Osteoarthritis of the right knee, 20 years after medial and lateral meniscectomies.

Fig. 184 Varus deformity of the left knee.

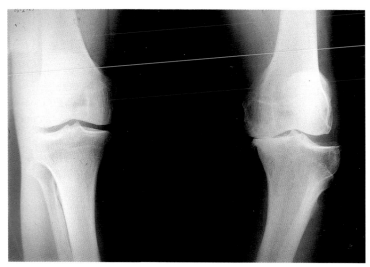

Fig. 185 OA of the medial compartment causing a varus deformity.

Heel bump

Synonyms

Winter heel; pump bump; Haglund syndrome.

Clinical features

Prominent thickening over the superolateral border of the calcaneum (Fig. 186). Usually seen in teenaged girls and both feet are affected.

Treatment

Pad beneath heel to minimize pressure from back of shoe.
  Spontaneous improvement is common and surgical treatment by calcaneal trimming or osteotomy is rarely necessary.

Rupture of calcaneal tendon

Clinical features

May occur in athletes or, more commonly, middle-aged people during activities such as dancing. Often a palpable gap in the tendon. When the calf on the affected side is squeezed the foot fails to plantar flex (Fig. 187).

Treatment

Surgical repair or rest in plaster with the foot in a plantar-flexed position.

Plantar fasciitis

Discomfort beneath the calcaneum at the attachment of the plantar fascia. Sometimes it occurs in inflammatory arthropathies but often no cause is found.

Clinical features

The pain is aggravated by weight bearing. Clinical examination is negative apart from local tenderness. A heel spur (Fig. 188) is often seen on radiographs, but is a common finding in asymptomatic people and is of no significance.

Treatment

Doughnut heel pad, local anaesthetic and steroid injection, ultrasound therapy. The condition settles spontaneously but may take some months.

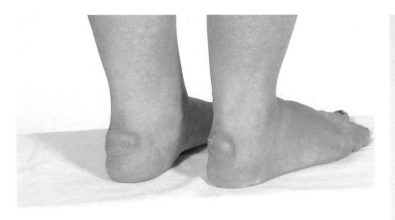

Fig. 186 Heel bumps.

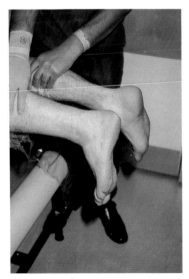

Fig. 187 Calf squeeze test. Rupture of left calcaneal tendon.

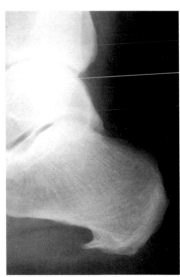

Fig. 188 Heel spur. An incidental finding in plantar fasciitis.

Talipes equinovarus

A congenital deformity in which the foot points downwards and is twisted inwards. The cause is unknown although there may be a family history. A similar deformity can occur in spina bifida and arthrogryphosis (p. 27).

Synonym

Club foot.

Clinical features

The deformity, which is obvious at birth, may be unilateral and bilateral (Fig. 189). The foot cannot be dorsiflexed to touch the front of the shin and there is often a deep skin crease on the medial border of the sole (Fig. 190).

Treatment

Neonatal. Treatment should start as soon as possible because the foot will rapidly stiffen in the position of deformity. The foot is initially strapped in the corrected position. Serial correcting plasters are used as the child grows.

Later. If full correction cannot be achieved by strapping, or if there has been no early treatment, surgical release of tight tissues will be necessary.

Talipes calcaneovalgus

A congenital condition in which the foot points upwards and is twisted outwards (Fig. 191). It is usually attributable to position *in utero* but may be caused by neurological conditions such as spina bifida.

Treatment

Unlike talipes equinovarus, the deformity improves spontaneously as the infant begins to move the legs freely, provided there is no underlying neurological abnormality. Corrective splintage is seldom needed.

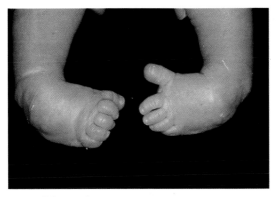

Fig. 189 Talipes equinovarus.

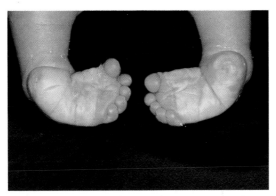

Fig. 190 Talipes equinovarus.

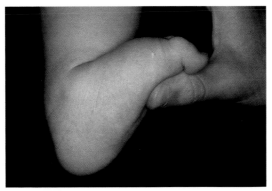

Fig. 191 Talipes calcaneovalgus.

Metatarsus adductus

A common condition in which the anterior part of the foot is deviated medially (Fig. 192), causing the child to walk with an intoeing gait.

Clinical features

Affects children aged 2–8. The foot can be corrected passively into the normal position. Physical examination will distinguish between metatarsus adductus and femoral anteversion (p. 109) which is another common cause of intoeing.

Treatment

In the majority of children the appearance improves without active treatment, although it may take some years.

Pes cavus

Accentuation of the longitudinal arch of the foot.

Causes

Idiopathic, familial or associated with neurological disorders such as poliomyelitis (p. 23), spina bifida (p. 27) and peroneal muscular atrophy (p. 29).

Clinical features

May be unilateral or bilateral, depending on the cause. Pes cavus is usually apparent in childhood and is obvious on examination (Fig. 193). Clawing of the toes (p. 141) is almost always present. In older children and adults there may be pain associated with callosities on the toes and under the metatarsal heads.

Treatment

Appropriate footwear and support insoles. If the deformity is severe the foot can be corrected by soft tissue release in childood, but in adults it is necessary to remove a wedge of bone to gain correction. Claw toes can be corrected surgically (p. 141).

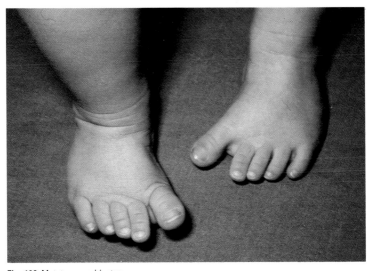

Fig. 192 Metatarsus adductus.

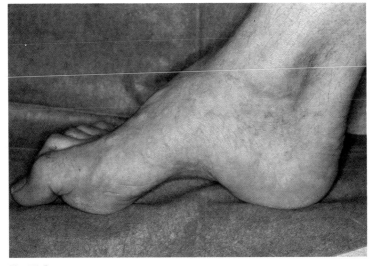

Fig. 193 Pes cavus.

Flat foot (pes planus)

In this common condition the medial border of the foot is in contact with the ground when standing (Fig. 194). Often the whole foot appears to have rotated into eversion around its longitudinal axis.

Two main types are recognized: mobile and rigid.

Mobile flat foot

Clinical features

The longitudinal arch is fully restored when standing on tiptoe. Symptoms are usually absent or mild. There may be some aching in the foot, and the shoes may wear rapidly on the inner border.

Treatment

An inner arch raise insole may be helpful symptomatically but the appearance is usually permanent. Surgical treatment is rarely needed.

Rigid flat foot

Clinical features

The longitudinal arch is not restored when standing on tiptoe. Often caused by a bony bridge (synostosis or bar) between two of the tarsal bones. Talocalcaneal and calcaneonavicular bars (Fig. 195) are most common.

Typically there is pain and limitation of movement in the foot—around the age of 12. There may be protective spasm of the peroneal muscles, hence the term 'peroneal spastic flat foot' is often applied to this condition (Fig. 196).

Radiographs show the bar, but special views or CT scan may be needed.

Treatment

Resection of the bar if feasible. Arthrodesis of the subtalar and midtarsal joints (triple fusion) may be necessary for secondary osteoarthritic changes.

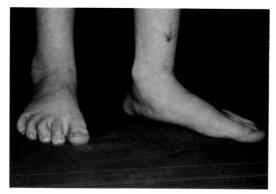

Fig. 194 Flat feet.

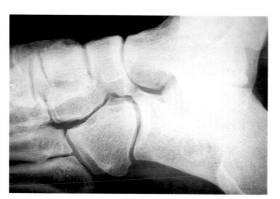

Fig. 195 A calcaneonavicular bar.

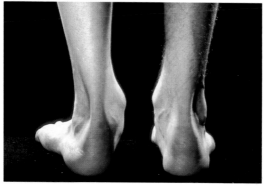

Fig. 196 Peroneal spasm affecting the left foot.

Osteochondritis

Navicular bone
Collapse of the centre of ossification in the bone. Like osteochondritis of other bones it is thought to be due to a disturbance of the blood supply.

Synonym

Köhler's disease.

Clinical features

Affects children aged 3–5. The child may complain of pain and be noticed to limp. Radiographs show compression and sometimes fragmentation of the centre of ossification (Fig. 197).

Treatment

Resolves spontaneously in a year or two. Rest in a cast for a few weeks may be necessary if there is severe pain.

Metatarsal head
Deformity of the second (occasionally third) metatarsal head possibly caused by interruption in the blood supply due to injury.

Synonym

Freiberg's infraction.

Clinical features

Affects teenagers. There is pain on walking. On examination there may be soft tissue swelling around the affected joint. Radiographs confirm the diagnosis (Fig. 198).

Treatment

Indicated only if pain is severe.

Early stages. Rest in cast.

Late cases. Excision arthroplasty is occasionally indicated.

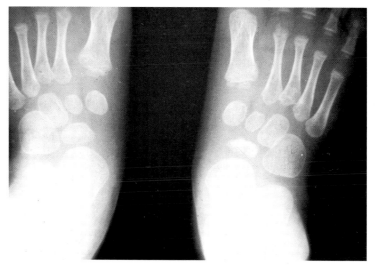

Fig. 197 Osteochondritis of navicular bone, right foot.

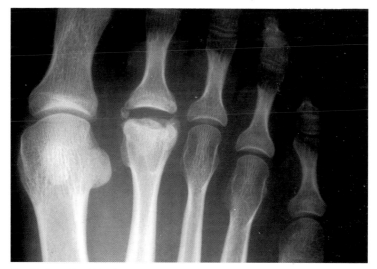

Fig. 198 Osteochondritis of second metatarsal head.

Syndactyly

Like syndactyly in the hand (p. 91), syndactyly in the foot may involve skin alone (Fig. 199), or may be complex and associated with multiple digital anomalies.

Treatment

Unlike the hand, the function of the foot is not affected by syndactyly and surgical correction is not indicated.

Overriding little toe

Synonym

Digitus quintus varus.

Clinical features

A fairly common congenital anomaly (Fig. 200). The deformity can be corrected passively at first. However, it does not improve spontaneously and may become fixed and subject to pressure from shoes.

Treatment

Surgical correction is usually necessary.

Underriding toes

A varus curvature of the lesser toes, usually most marked in the third and fourth (Fig. 201). There is often a family history.

Synonyms

Curly toes; varus toes.

Clinical features

The toes function normally and some spontaneous improvement in the appearance is common.

Treatment

Seldom needed. In severe cases the alignment of the toes can be improved by transferring the flexor tendon into the extensor tendon around the lateral border of the toe.

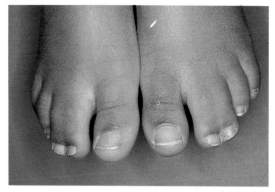

Fig. 199 Syndactyly between second and third toes.

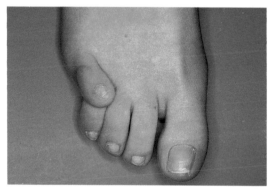

Fig. 200 Overriding fifth toe

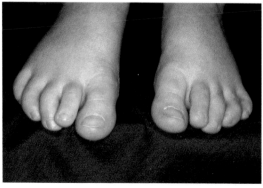

Fig. 201 Underriding toes.

Hammer toe

Fixed flexion deformity of the proximal interphalangeal joint of one of the lesser toes. It may be an isolated deformity or associated with hallux valgus (p. 143) (Fig. 202). A painful callosity often forms on the dorsum of the affected joint.

Treatment

Local pad to relieve pressure or arthrodesis of the affected joint in a straight position.

Mallet toe

Fixed flexion of the terminal interphalangeal joint of one of the lesser toes (Fig. 203). A painful callosity often forms on the pulp of the affected toe.

Treatment

As for hammer toe (see above).

Claw toes

Flexion of the interphalangeal joints and extension of the metatarsophalangeal joints of one or, more commonly, several of the lesser toes (Fig. 204). It is caused by an imbalance of the intrinsic and extrinsic muscles acting on the toes and often associated with pes cavus (p. 133). The deformity may be idiopathic or caused by any condition that can affect muscle function in the foot, e.g. spina bifida (p. 27), poliomyelitis (p. 23), peroneal muscular atrophy (p. 29) and ischaemia.

Treatment

Shoes should have adequate room to avoid pressure on toes. Surgical correction is by tendon transfer if the deformity is mobile, or arthrodesis if it is fixed.

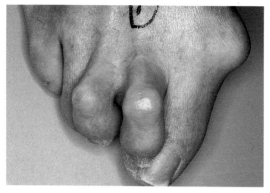

Fig. 202 Hammer toe deformity in second and third toes.

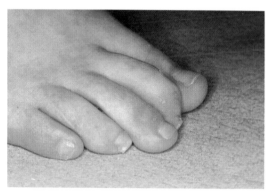

Fig. 203 Mallet toe deformity in second toe.

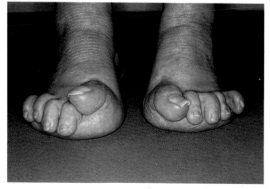

Fig. 204 Clawing of toes.

Hallux valgus

In this condition the great toe is excessively deviated towards the second toe and may come to lie over or under it.

Cause

Unknown. There is often a strong family history. Wearing tight pointed shoes may aggravate the deformity but probably does not cause it.

Clinical features

A common condition of middle-aged and elderly women. The patient complains of pressure over the prominent head of the first metatarsal bone (the 'bunion') or the second toe. An inflamed bursa may form over the first metatarsal head (Fig. 205). The metatarsal heads often spread out, causing widening of the foot. Painful callosities can develop under the metatarsal heads (Fig. 207). Shoe fitting is a problem. Radiographs confirm the diagnosis and sometimes demonstrate that the second toe has dislocated at the metatarsophalangeal joint (Fig. 206).

Treatment

Conservative. Comfortable shoes and protection of pressure areas.

Surgical. Many operations have been described, but the results are not always satisfactory. In young people the great toe can be realigned by osteotomy of the first metatarsal bone. In older patients arthrodesis or excision arthroplasty (Keller's arthroplasty) of the first metatarsophalangeal joint are preferred.

Realigning the big toe will not relieve pain from plantar callosities, which is often the major complaint. If an inappropriate operation is performed, the results of surgery will be unsatisfactory.

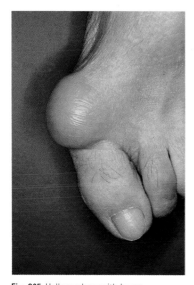

Fig. 205 Hallux valgus with bursa.

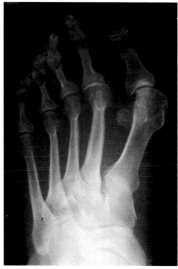

Fig. 206 Hallux valgus.

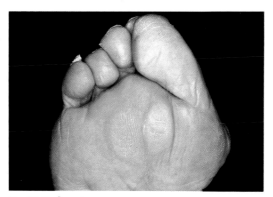

Fig. 207 Plantar callosities associated with hallux valgus.

Hallux rigidus

Osteoarthritis of the metatarsophalangeal joint at the base of the great toe. Probably secondary to previous minor trauma.

Clinical features

Equally common in men and women. Unlike OA in other joints, hallux rigidus often affects young people in their 30s.

There is discomfort in the joint, especially when the toe is dorsiflexed, e.g. when 'toeing-off' from the ground during walking. On examination there is often a visible dorsomedial osteophyte, over which a bursa may form (Fig. 208). Passive dorsiflexion of the joint is limited (Fig. 210).

Radiographs show typical changes of OA, with loss of joint space, osteophytes and sclerosis of subchondral bone (Fig. 209).

Treatment

Conservative. Comfortable shoes. A bar on the sole of the shoe under the metatarsal heads will prevent painful dorsiflexion of the great toe but is rather clumsy in practice.

Surgical. For severe symptoms only. The options include arthrodesis of the joint or interpositional arthroplasty using a silicone rubber spacer. In older patients Keller's operation (p. 143) may be used.

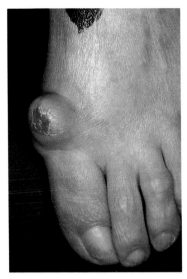

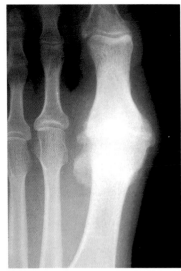

Fig. 208 Hallux rigidus. Bursa over dorsal osteophyte.

Fig. 209 Radiographic appearance of hallux rigidus.

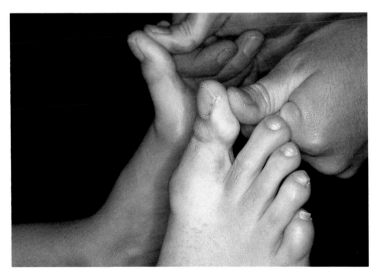

Fig. 210 Hallux rigidus. Limited dorsiflexion of right great toe.

Bunionette

Prominence of the fifth metatarsal head. Often associated with an overlying bursa or callosity.

Synonym   Tailor's bunion.

Clinical features   Most often seen in teenaged girls. It is usually bilateral (Fig. 211), and causes difficulty in shoe fitting.

Treatment   Symptoms are usually relieved by wearing broader shoes. Surgical treatment by osteotomy of the metatarsal neck or excision of the metatarsal head is rarely needed.

Accessory bones

These are common in the foot. Generally speaking they are of no significance but may be mistaken for fractures on radiographs and can sometimes cause local prominences in the foot. They are usually bilateral.

Examples are:

Os trigonum.   Lies behind the talus and above the calcaneum. Sometimes attached to one of these bones (Fig. 212).

Os tibiale externum.   Lies on the medial border of the foot in association with the navicular bone (Fig. 213). Sometimes associated with a mobile flat foot (p. 135) due to an abnormal insertion of the tendon of tibialis posterior.

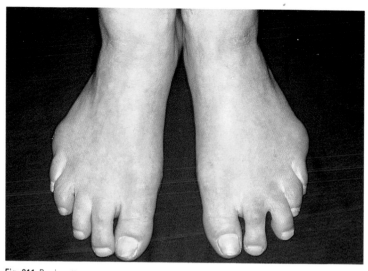

Fig. 211 Bunionettes.

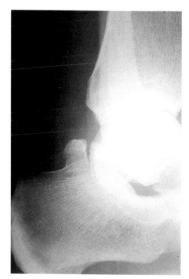

Fig. 212 An os trigonum attached to the calcaneum.

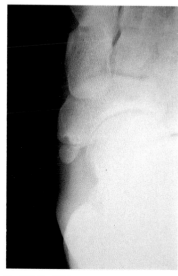

Fig. 213 Os tibiale externum.

Plantar interdigital neuroma

A fibrous thickening of the interdigital nerve between the third and fourth metatarsal heads. Not a true neuroma but may be due to local ischaemia or entrapment.

Synonym

Morton's neuroma.

Clinical features

Affects middle-aged women predominantly. The complaint is of burning, neuritic pain passing into the third and fourth toes after standing or walking. It is often eased by taking off the shoe and rubbing the foot.

On examination there is seldom any abnormality, but sometimes there is tenderness over the site of the 'neuroma' (Fig. 214) and discomfort may be elicited by squeezing the forefoot from either side.

Treatment

A metatarsal pad will spread out the bones and relieve local pressure. If it is not successful, surgical removal of the lesion (Fig. 215) will relieve the discomfort. The loss of sensation between the toes does not cause a problem.

Plantar fibromatosis

In this condition a nodule or nodules forms within the plantar fascia.

Clinical features

A rather uncommon condition that can occur in childhood or adult life. In adults it may be associated with Dupuytren's disease of the hand (p. 95) or can occur as an isolated condition.

Treatment

Excision may be necessary if the lesions are large (Fig. 216) or their nature is in doubt. However, surgery should be avoided if possible as troublesome recurrence is almost always the rule in adults.

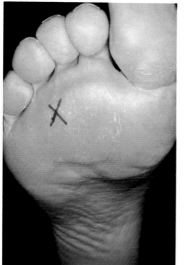

Fig. 214 Interdigital neuroma. Site of discomfort.

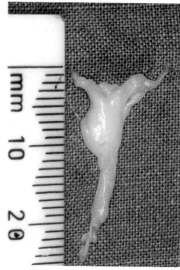

Fig. 215 An excised 'neuroma'.

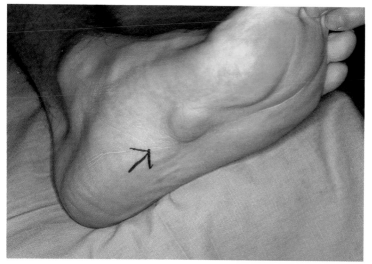

Fig. 216 Plantar fibromatosis.

Onychogryposis

Thickened deformed nails.

Clinical features

The big toe is most often affected (Fig. 217). Usually a result of poor personal hygiene and most often seen in elderly people who are unable to look after themselves.

Treatment

Regular care of the nails by a chiropodist. If regrowth is a problem, the germinal matrix of the nail should be ablated surgically.

Subungual exostosis

A bony outgrowth from the terminal phalanx of the great toe. May be associated with chronic infection around the nail.

Clinical features

Usually affects young people. The exostosis causes the nail to be raised from its bed. Local granulation tissue (Fig. 218) causes discomfort. Radiographs will show the bony prominence (Fig. 219).

Treatment

Surgical excision.

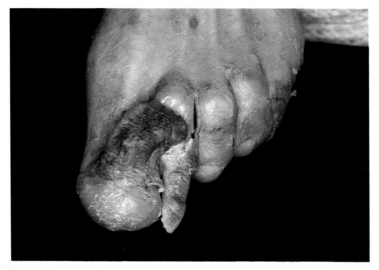

Fig. 217 Onychogryposis.

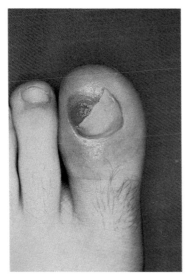

Fig. 218 Subungual exostosis.

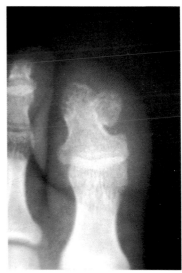

Fig. 219 Subungual exostosis.

Index